Gérald Ubassy
Shape and Color
The Key to Successful Ceramic Restorations

Shape and Color

The Key to Successful Ceramic Restorations

Gérald Ubassy

Dental technician, Avignon, France

Quintessence Publishing Co, Inc
Chicago, Berlin, London, São Paulo, and Tokyo

Title of the Original French Edition:
Formes et couleurs — Les clés du succès en céramique dentaire
© 1992 by Quintessenz Verlags-GmbH, Berlin
© Editions CdP, Paris, 1992

For Landry

Library of Congress Cataloging-in-Publication Data

Ubassy, Gérald.
    [Formen und Farben. English]
    Shape and color : the key to successful ceramic restorations /
Gérald Ubassy.
        p. cm.
    Includes bibliographical references and index.
    ISBN 0-86715-207-9
    1. Dental ceramics. 2. Fillings (Dentistry) 3. Inlays
(Dentistry) 4. Dentistry--Aesthetics. I. Title.
        [DNLM: 1. Dental Restoration, Permanent. 2. Dental Porcelain.
3. Ceramics. 4. Estetics, Dental. WU   190   U12f   1993a]
RK655, U2313   1993
617.6'95--dc20
DNLM/DLC
for Library of Congress   93-1039
                                                               CIP

quinte//ence
book/

Copyright © 1993 by Quintessence Publishing Co, Inc.

Lithography: Toppan Printing Co., (H.K.) Ltd., Hong Kong
Typesetting, Printing, and Binding: Bosch-Druck, Landshut/Ergolding

ISBN 0-86715-207-9

Contents

Preface

The development of new techniques and materials enables the contemporary dental technician to satisfy even those patients who are particularly concerned about the esthetics of their teeth. Because of this legitimate expectation, our profession must keep consistently informed and must exchange information. Thus the basic thought that kept me motivated while completing this textbook was the strong desire for "communication" – a keyword and characteristic of a progressive profession.

This book is dedicated especially to those technicians who apply our methods in practice. Clinical aspects are part of every chapter in order to imbue the described methods with necessary pertinence and reliability.

Another keyword of our book is *observation*, which is the basis of my work, and nature as a most important "keyhole."

The study of shapes and microshapes and how they interact with color is the guideline of this book. These studies are of utmost importance to me.

On the other hand, I abolished concepts that are all-too-rigid and that merely stereotype artificial teeth. This influenced me to take into consideration characteristics such as gender, personality, morphology, and the character of the patient. Artificial teeth should definitely reflect all these parameters and include the finest detail regarding shape and microshape as a contribution to perfect integration of dental restorations.

It is obvious that periodontal conditions as well as functional aspects must be considered while striving for form, color, and esthetics because they stand for long-lasting success.

Consequently, I envisage an ideal where a dental restoration is not only represented by its name and function but even more so by its appearance.

None of this can be accomplished, however, without close collaboration on the concept and the goal, or without excellent interpersonal contact between dentist and dental technician.

This book is highly illustrated because diagrams and photographs represent the best explanation for many techniques.

Finally, I admonish the reader to remember that all results should be questioned over and over if we are to progress beyond our current possibilities and knowledge.

Gérald Ubassy

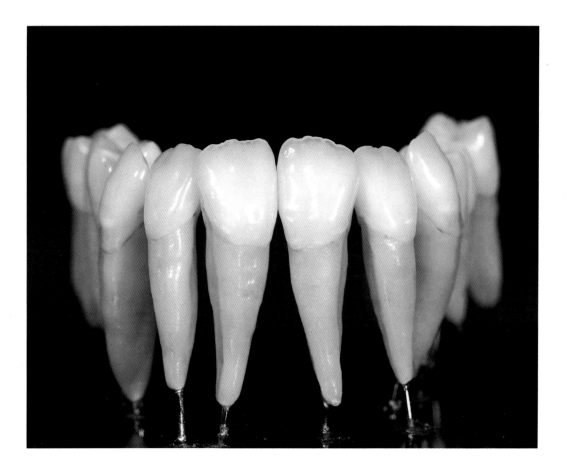

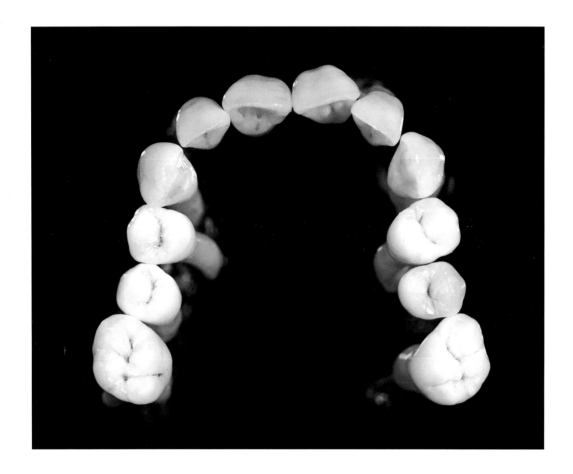

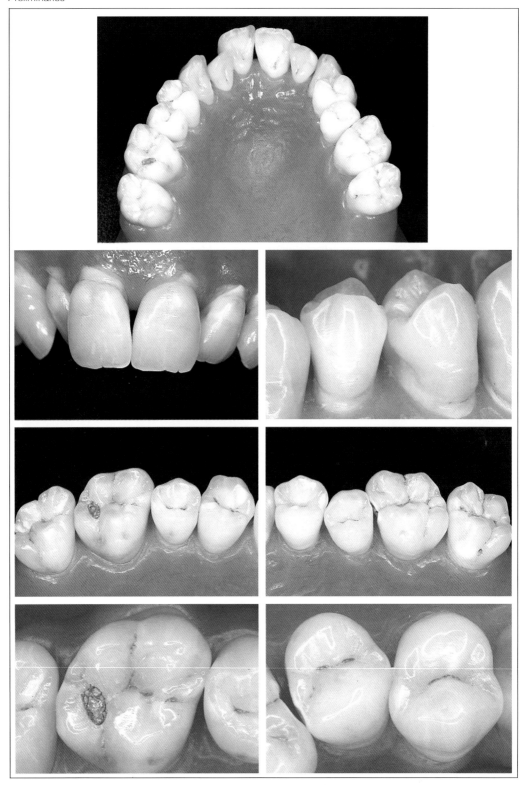

Acknowledgments

Completion of this book demanded many hours of work as well as moral and technical support.

I am most pleased to have the opportunity to thank all those who contributed to the publication of this book.

First of all I thank my wife, Helen, who has always been a constructive critic owing to her patience and sensitivity as well as her natural sense for esthetics; her technical assistance during preparation of the manuscript was always appreciated.

I thank *André Moreau,* who teaches at the School of Dental Technology, Montpellier, who was able to impart his knowledge and his devotion to us, his students.

Special thanks to Ivoclar and in particular to my friend Herbert Frick for the technical help and attention they contributed.

My gratitude to all my customers with whom I have developed strong professional as well as extraordinary personal relations. Skillful work of superb quality cannot be performed with an adequate laboratory team; here I must mention my friends and colleagues: Jean-Marie Milesi and Jean-François Zalejski, both devoted and outstanding dental technicians.

The acknowledgments would be incomplete without thanks to the publishers Quintessence and H.W. Haase for the confidence they showed by encouraging me to write this book.

Foreword

In recent years there has been no shortage of publications dealing with dental ceramics. The indisputable superiority of this biomaterial over any other cosmetic material, and the most recent developments in this field of metal ceramic restorations without metal substructures, have influenced clinical researchers as well as dental technicians to strive for a realistic, even artistic use of dental ceramics.

In their books, however, ceramists often tend to describe modeling methods or their build-up technique without communicating a clear or comprehensive view to the reader about this subject.

If we try to mimic nature from now on – without the claim to do it even better but ambitious nevertheless to achieve equal results – there is only one rule to follow: **observation.** And if there were only one term to keep in mind after reading Gérald Ubassy's book, this would be the one.

In the sun- and light-dominated region of Provence where Ubassy was born, he developed powers of observation that deserve more than just attention: modesty and patience.

Natural teeth vary greatly in color and shape. They reveal ample information about the background and personality of our patients.

Modern dental ceramics also demand interest in the individual as technical know-how, and Ubassy makes it obvious in his book. He clearly explains in a sensitive way how to treat each patient individually in order to observe and understand precisely the means of color, its value, texture of surfaces, and the condi-

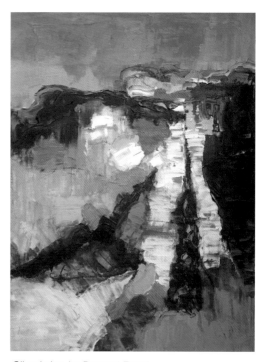

Oil painting by Bernard Touati.

tion of adjacent soft tissues. Eventually, in his honest ways, he merely hands over the keys for success.

Rarely has there been a book about dental ceramics so complete without being superficial: it covers how to polish ceramic, create fissures, fabricate working casts in the laboratory. All that is apparently of subordinate significance is marvelous. Without exaggerating, no compromise in creating a restoration will be necessary if thorough observation is the guideline.

A dental ceramist will only mature, if he or she respects details and strives for perfection. Every illustration in this book gives evidence of the methodical quest for naturalness and beauty. Ubassy depicts vividly new fields such as ceramic inlays and onlays and leucite-reinforced all-ceramic crowns. These resin-retained restorations introduce new and seemingly successful solutions in prosthodontics. Few books can describe so vividly and convincingly the necessary laboratory procedures like Ubassy's.

There is no doubt about it: Ubassy shines in every chapter of this book. His inborn sense for adaptation and his enthusiasm for the new provide his work with some of the highest esthetic qualities I have ever feasted my eyes on. And sometimes it seems to me as if I were contemplating a beautiful picture . . .

Bernard Touati

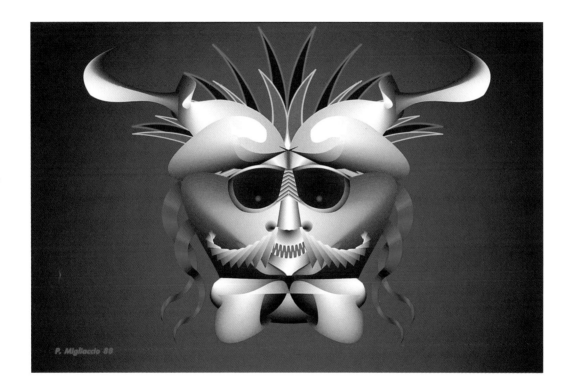

P. Migliaccio 88

Several illustrations are included in this book that have nothing to do with our profession. These pictures have been created with the assistence of computers.

Let me now introduce Pietro Migliaccio, the artist who created such artistic work that is surrealistic, baroque, and abstract – all at the same time. Pietro, in his own brilliant ways, is capable of playing with shape and color. But most of all I believe that with these computer drawings he indicates a strong and miraculous connection between art and technology if it is performed with like perfection.

1 Basic Terms of the Phenomenon of Color

In 1676, the physicist Isaac Newton performed an experiment that showed that a single ray of white light can be broken up into the colors of the spectrum when made to pass through a crystal prism. This spectrum includes all basic colors except purple. Newton performed the experiment as follows (Fig 1-1): a ray of light passing through an aperture strikes the prism. The "white" light, now passing through the prism, is separated into the colors of the spectrum. These bands of colors can be projected on a screen, thereby creating a spectrum too. The spectrum spreads uninterruptedly from red through orange, yellow, green, and blue to violet. If the separated bands of color are further collected through a lens, this addition process will result in "white" light on a second screen. Thus, the spectrum is a result of *refraction* of light.

Colors originate from lightwaves, which represent a specific type of electromagnetic energy. The human eye can only perceive light ranging from 400 to 700 mµ. Wavelengths are measured in microns:
- 1 micron   = 1 µm = 1/1,000 mm
- 1 millimicron = 1 mµ = 1/1,000,000 mm

Wavelengths of the spectral colors and the number of oscillations per second are:

Color	Wavelength	No. of oscillations
Red	800 – 650 mµ	400 – 470 trillion
Orange	640 – 590 mµ	470 – 520 trillion
Yellow	580 – 550 mµ	520 – 590 trillion
Green	530 – 490 mµ	590 – 650 trillion
Blue	480 – 460 mµ	650 – 700 trillion
Indigo	450 – 440 mµ	700 – 760 trillion
Violet	430 – 390 mµ	760 – 800 trillion

The ratio of oscillation from red to violet is approximately 1 : 2, similar to that of an octave. Every spectral color is specified by wavelength and the number of oscillations. Lightwaves are colorless; color is created in our eyes and brains.

The physicist Young later performed Newton's experiment conversely. Whereas Newton broke up light into its spectral colors using a crystal prism, Young put them together again. He made the separated rays of light converge and so regained the "white" light.

In order to understand this physical phenomenon (ie, the fact that several bright colors, which sometimes become darker by mixing, result in a lighter color) we must remember that all these colors are fractions of "white" light; colors that are generated by rays of light that merely reproduce the effects of light. That means if we combine one so-called light-mixture or light-color with another, the result will be a more intense and lighter color. The sum of the combination green, and red must consequently yield a lighter color — yellow in this case.

In addition, Young proved something significant regarding our studies: while experimenting with his color lanterns, he found out by elimination that the spectral colors for the same spectrum can be reduced to three basic colors. We can "reconstruct" "white" light by combining the colors red, green, and blue (Fig 1-2). He mixed two out of the three and the result was the other three: blue, purple or magenta, and yellow. All in all he specified *primary* and *secondary* colors of the spectrum:

- **Primary spectral colors:**
  - Red
  - Green
  - Blue

- **Secondary spectral colors:**
  (mixing of two primary colors)
  - blue light + green light = cyan (1)
  - red light + blue light = purple (2)
  - green light + red light = yellow

(1) Cyan: technical term for that secondary color. The hue of cyan is identical with a neutral blue of medium intensity.
(2) Purple: or magenta is identical with a carmine of medium hue.

The previous classification of spectral colors enables us to specify those colors that are complementary to certain other spectral colors. The secondary colors lack only one primary color to appear as complementary color and to recompose the "white" light (and vice versa).

- **Complementary colors:**
  - Yellow is complementary to indigo
  - Cyan is complementary to red
  - Purple is complementary to green

Absorption and Reflection

Imagine: all that surrounds you, every object you can see, is receiving the three primary colors: blue, red, and green. Some of these objects reflect all of the light they receive, whereas others absorb it totally or almost totally. But most of them absorb partially and reflect the rest. Thus the natural law is:

- Opaque objects that are exposed to light reflect all or a certain part of the light they receive.

As yet it is not fully understood why we perceive color and relate to a particular one as, eg, red. Why are tomatoes red? What we know is that if light strikes this tomato it receives all three primary colors: blue, green, and red (Fig 1-3, *C*).

Even the page you are reading right now absorbs these three invisible colors of light (blue, green, and red), and the way the paper receives the light colors are returned. The object reflects the colors and the sum of all three is white, the color of the paper (Fig 1-3, *A*).

If the object struck by light is a pot of India ink, the exact opposite will happen: the three primary colors strike the pot but will be fully absorbed, thus leaving the object unchanged; it appears black to us (Fig 1-3, *B*).

If light strikes a banana, again the three primary colors are received. The banana absorbs the blue and reflects the green and red components. Red and green combined yields yellow (Fig 1-3, *D*). Take a plum: it absorbs green and reflects red and blue, giving the plum its purple appearance (Fig 1-3, *E*).

Light, Color, and Pigments in Dental Porcelain

We are just about to delve into dental ceramics. This material consists of colored powder and pigments with which we try to imitate the phenomena of light and color previously explained. We will learn to understand the way color acts to enable this imitation.

We have seen that light, while "coloring" objects exposed to its influence, uses three colors — bright and dark ones. Mixing of two

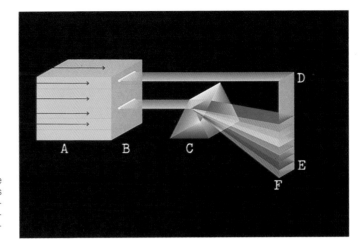

Fig 1-1 Light is broken up into the colors of the spectrum when it is passed through a prism. *(A)* sunlight, *(B)* lenses, *(C)* prism, *(D)* without prism, *(E)* with prism, *(F)* spectrum.

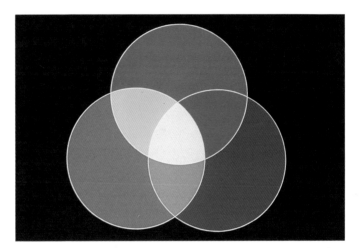

Fig 1-2 Primary colors of the spectrum. Synthesis through addition. Overlapping of all three recomposes the "white" light.

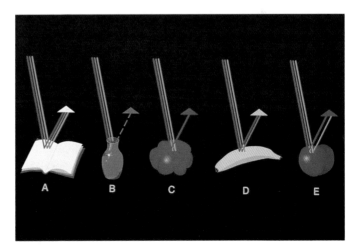

Fig 1-3 Absorption and reflection. Opaque objects that are exposed to light reflect all or a certain part of the light they receive.

produces another three, lighter colors, and finally mixing all colors together recomposes the "white" light. As far as we are concerned, however, we cannot "paint" with light.

In the field of dental ceramics it is not possible to obtain lighter colors by means of mixing darker colors as is done in painting.

Additive and Subtractive Syntheses

When painting pictures we learn that combinations of colors change depending on what has been omitted from light, ie, we always work from lighter colors to darker colors. For instance, if you mix red and green you obtain the darker color brown. And if you mix cyan with purple and yellow (three very bright colors) you will get black. This is precisely the reverse to the combination of spectral colors.

Thus, when light "paints" an object it is adding light rays of different colors: the colors are produced by addition or *additive synthesis*.

When we work with colors in dental ceramics, we subtract light; we obtain these colors by means of subtraction or *subtractive synthesis*.

How does light "paint" (Fig 1-2)?:

– *Additive synthesis:* to produce the secondary color yellow, red and green are mixed: such mixture yields a lighter color, a brighter light. Yellow represents the sum or additive synthesis of red and green.

How do pigments "paint" (Fig 1-4)?:

– *Subtractive synthesis:* to produce the secondary color green, we have to mix cyan and yellow. Regarding spectral colors, blue absorbs red and yellow absorbs blue. The only color that reflects both of them is green, which is therefore subtracted out from blue and red.

After having investigated provenance and origin of colors we are in possession of a fundamental knowledge that enables us to describe the entire polychromy of colors in a diagram (Fig 1-5).

Below is the classification of primary, secondary, and tertiary pigments:

● **Primary pigments:**
  ○ Cyan
  ○ Purple (magenta)
  ○ Yellow

Primary colors are those that cannot be produced by mixing others; they are the original colors that can be combined to make all the other colors of nature.

● **Secondary pigments:**
  ○ Orange-red
  ○ Green
  ○ Indigo

These secondary colors can be obtained by mixing the above-mentioned primary colors according to Fig 1-4.

If we mix secondary and primary colors, a different, darker tone will be obtained, representing a tertiary color, and so forth. In this way we can produce innumerable nuances, all deriving from the primary pigments (cyan, purple or magenta, and yellow).

The Language of Colors

Conveying information about what we see is an intricate process because the human visual system depends on interpretation.

If we describe an object by means of two of its characteristics, in this case shape and color, the object may appear to be relatively simple when we talk about tangible dimensions such as height, length, and width. However, for most of us it will prove a very difficult task to describe an object's exact color, because it has never occurred to many of us that color, too, is a three-dimensional phenomenon. Therefore, remarks like "darken with yellow" or "gently lighten" apparently give evidence of how little is known about this phenomenon.

Anyone wanting to work intelligently with dental ceramics must know about the dimen-

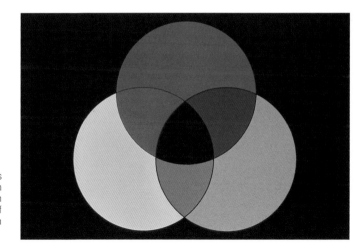

Fig 1-4 When working with colors we subtract from light and we obtain these colors by means of subtraction or subtractive synthesis. Mixing of the three primary colors in a certain ratio produces black.

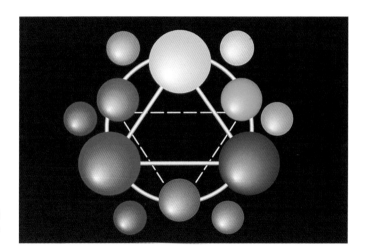

Fig 1-5 Polychromy of colors that are classified in primary (or basic), secondary, and tertiary.

sions of colors. Otherwise he or she will be entangled in an awkward system of trial-and-error while attempting to find the appropriate color match.

Albert Henri Munsell's contribution to the understanding of colors is relatively recent. It was in 1915 when his *Atlas of the* Munsell *Color System* was published. He describes color as a three-dimensional phenomenon and compares it to the body of an ashlar. Whereas all colors in this atlas are arranged in subsequent order, the three-dimensional model is similar to the shape of an irregular

ball (Fig 1-6). The three dimensions of color are hue, brilliance (value), and saturation (chroma).

– *Hue* is the quality that distinguishes one family of colors from another, eg, red from yellow or green from blue. If we say, for instance, that a tooth looks yellow or orange, we are describing its hue.

– *Value* or *brilliance* is the quality by which we distinguish a light color from a dark one. It is represented by the achromatic axis in the center of Munsell's cylinder, where white is at the top and black at the

21

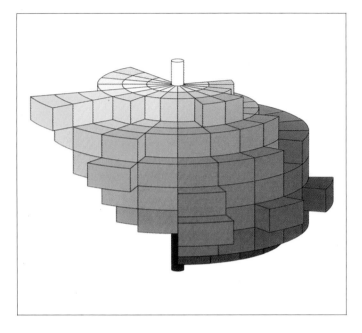

Fig 1-6 Three-dimensional classification of colors by Henri Munsell.

bottom (Fig 1-6). There is a scale of grays ranging gradually from black to white and thus connecting the two extremes. Black has zero brilliance whereas white shows maximum brilliance.
– *Chroma* or *saturation* is the quality by which we distinguish a strong color from a weak one. For example: one tooth may look more yellow or orange than another.

It is so difficult to describe color strictly visually that dictionaries are filled with hundreds of names of colors all meant to depict objects. Some of these names are more, others less, familiar. The expression a "green apple" may act as a graphic example, but everyone has a different idea what this is supposed to mean.

To specify color it would be more precise to refer to a tone that we use as standard. The discrepancies can then be described by means of hue, brilliance, and saturation in accordance to the *Munsell* system (Fig 1-6). Brilliance is the most important of the three dimensions of color. If the hue of a restoration matches the adjacent teeth but its brilliance is

too dominant, the result will inevitably appear artificial. There is a simple method to alter (ie, decrease) the brilliance of ceramic without coloring the surface. This method will be discussed later (chapter 5: "The three-dimensional shade guide and changing brilliance of colors"). Conversely, if the hue is correct while brilliance is low, the restoration will appear gray.

Artificial teeth should be produced more realistically after the model, including all distinctions concerning hue and saturation of colors. If, for instance, canines are compared to the rest of the dentition they may show a different hue and more chroma. Because of reasons mentioned above, colors of differing brilliance should not be selected.

Few objects show as much visual differentiation as human teeth. It would be a serious error to focus solely on the hue even though "hue" and "color" are virtually on equal terms. What we should try to imitate is the appearance of a tooth that is the sum of all its visual dimensions. For example: a piece of wood and a piece of glass may be of

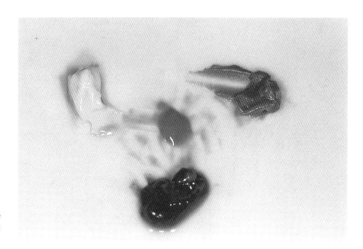

Fig 1-7 The composed gray in the center has been created by mixing the three primary colors.

identical color and still look completely different. The degree of translucency of a dental material is doubtless equally significant. Human teeth are characterized by degrees of translucency. The characteristic of a human tooth is mainly designated by its translucency; light penetrates the tooth and vanishes in the oral cavity. This is precisely the reason that makes the subject of "color" so complicated in dentistry. Therefore, provided color is used in relation to translucent objects, we may use four dimensions as definition: hue, saturation, brilliance, and the degree of translucency (see chapter 13: "Transparency and Translucency").

Simple and Complex Grays

If we relate to gray as pigmentation and not the degree of translucency, we will notice there are two kinds of grays: simple ones and composed ones. Simple grays contain black and white color pigments, whereas the composed grays are a combination of primary colors of which every component absorbs a particular part of the spectrum (Fig 1-7). The difference, for instance, is the fact that the composed grays can show a considerable degree of translucency while the color pigments are largely scattered in a transparent core. Simple grays, on the other hand, are inevitably opaque; there is no such thing as a transparent white color pigment. Staining colors in (dental) ceramics are mostly similar to coloring matter. All objects can be colored with any color except for white. Therefore, a simple gray will never be used for the adaptation of brilliance, particularly not on the surface of a translucent object, unless a "painted" object is the desired result.

It seems imperative that every dental ceramist have some basic knowledge about color before working with colors in dental ceramics. Furthermore, this basic knowledge will ensure improved ways of communication between the dentist and the dental technician.

2 Relation of Personality, Facial Esthetics, and Dentolabial Esthetics

It is incomprehensible that an extensive esthetic reconstruction of anterior teeth could be fabricated without the ceramist ever knowing the gender or age of the patient or without even having seen the patient before. Hence it is also improper to shape and arrange teeth identically for each and every patient. Frequently people can be seen in everyday life or on television with artificial teeth that do not match their personality. One of the major misconceptions in our profession is that a certain technological quality standard of a restoration suffices. There is a strong interaction between all aspects of esthetics, particularly concerning

- Personality
- Esthetics of facial structures
- Dentolabial esthetics

Hence, before one reconstructs a smile, one must briefly study different personalities and temperaments.

We are constantly striving to have access to maximum information; this may mean working from esthetic "schemes" of sets of teeth, as it used to be a few years ago. It can also mean using photographs, eg, an older picture of the patient's smile, a current photograph of the patient's face, even extracted teeth or old provisional restorations that simulate exactly the final shape of the planned restoration.

The most desirable information, of course, comes from seeing the patient and having a personal talk about his or her expectations and the professional's possibilities.

The following pictures illustrate successful restorative solutions that embody a harmonic balance between personality, facial esthetics, and dentolabial esthetics.

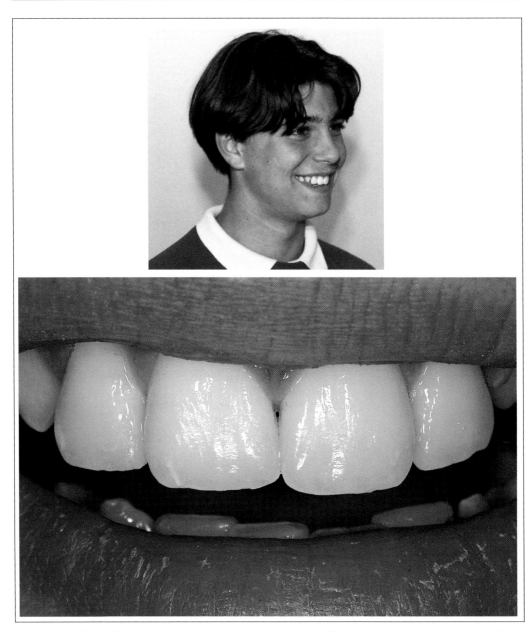

Figs 2-1 and 2-2 A 13-year-old boy who still has a mixed dentition. But the relation between his personality, his facial esthetics, and his teeth is already showing. Note the irregular surface texture of his teeth.

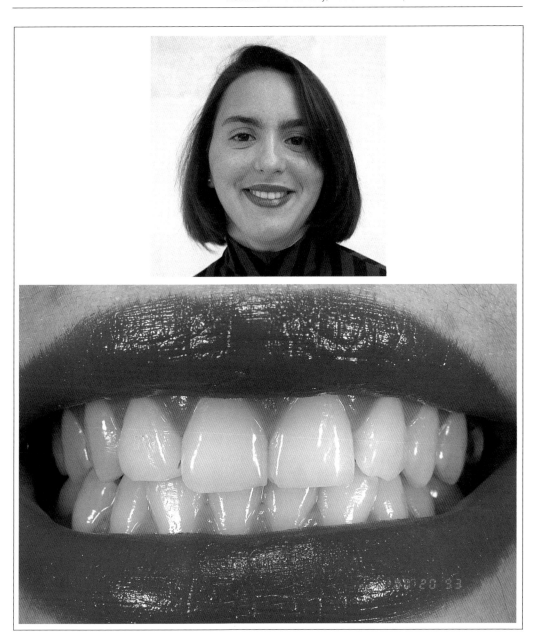

Figs 2-3 and 2-4 This patient's smile and her personality are in harmonic balance. Note that the smile is esthetic although the teeth are not aligned as regularly as piano keys; they show slight differences in position and variations in color.

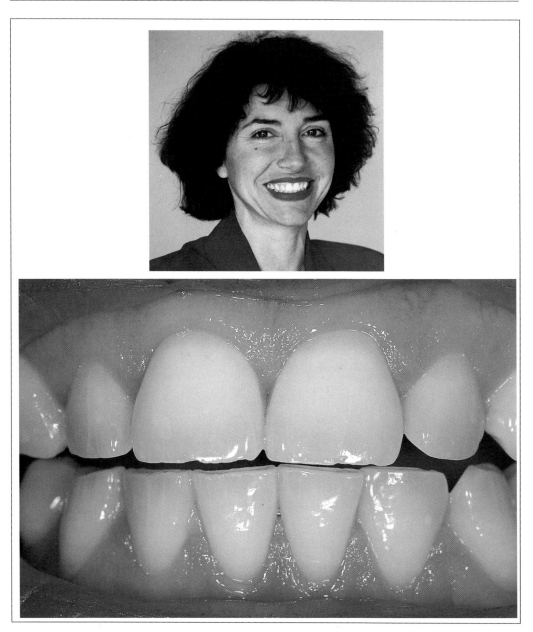

Figs 2-5 and 2-6 A smile that is conspicuous by its distinct tooth shape makes a strong personality recognizable. This pretty smile is in harmony with the face.

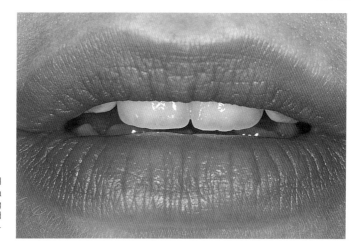

Fig 2-7 The visible line of incisal edges contributes significantly to a harmonic balance of a face. Nothing appears stern or rigid. Teeth 11 and 12 have been restored with all-ceramic crowns (Empress system).

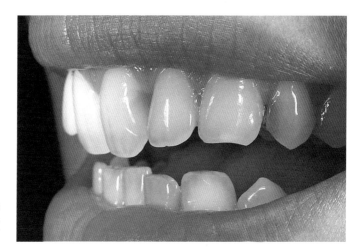

Fig 2-8 We must learn to observe teeth in each and every position. Side views are important for studying tooth shape and tooth axis.

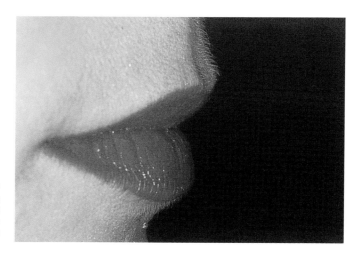

Fig 2-9 Lips are one of the major criteria of personality. Complete rehabilitation of anterior regions involves consideration about the balance between projection of the teeth and lip support.

ESTHETIC SUCCESS

TOOTH SHAPE

SURFACE STRUCTURE
(microshape and glaze)

COLOR OF TEETH

3   Colored Wax

A smile – an esthetic smile – can only be reconstructed successfully if thorough studies on wax models are used as a first step.

The use of dark red, green, or blue wax is common practice in many dental laboratories. If the wax differs in color from the working model and contrasts seemingly better with the lighter cast, however, perception of shape and its dimensions appears to be inaccurate. Absorption of light by dark objects reduces

our sight at the cost of detail and dimension (Fig 3-1).

Ivory-colored wax contrasts with dark wax to more suitably show contour, but too much reflection of the light-colored wax is detrimental for detail perception. Studies about the esthetics of a person's smile show less depth and seem to present only a two-dimensional image – not three-dimensional – as in a model of a three-dimensional space (Fig 3-2).

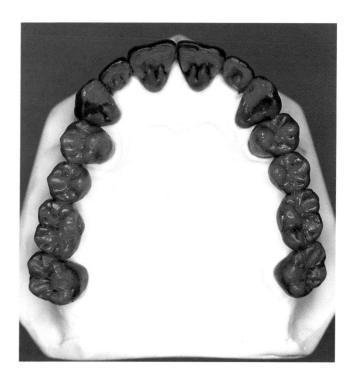

Fig 3-1 The visual perception of colors and its dimension is quite inaccurate if dark-colored wax is used. The absorption of light by dark objects reduces our visual abilities at the cost of details and real dimension of these objects.

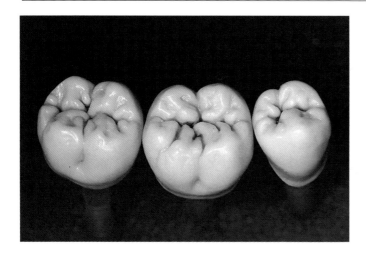

Fig 3-2 Ivory-colored wax contrasts with dark wax more suitably to show contour, but too much reflection of the light-colored wax is detrimental for detail perception: the objects appear "flat." The ivory-colored wax models have been fabricated by Jean-Marie Milesi.

Using colored wax enables us to reproduce the shades of natural teeth and eliminate the lack of perception by adding the three-dimensional aspect. So the uniformity of the shades of a monochromatic, ivory-colored wax is split (Figs 3-3 and 3-4).

Two advantages — educational and psychological — seem to favor the use of colored wax models.

Educational Advantages

The making of colored wax models can be coupled with step-by-step build-up of the ceramic, thus generating interest in studying and valuing color properly. Using wax models, it is possible to imitate desired effects and correct them without difficulty, making the fabrication of the final restoration easier for the future ceramist.

The build-up of artificial teeth can be studied methodically without being hindered by constant humidity as a precondition or the experience of undesirable shifts of the ceramic layers. To include the use of colored wax into the training of dental technicians

seems to me crucial. The similarities of the colors of wax and those of natural teeth improve the dental technician's knowledge about color and make vividly clear how color and shape interact. For the build-up of posterior teeth, colored wax is equally useful; three-dimensional occlusal concepts are easier to grasp (Fig 3-5). The first attempts will presumably take longer compared to working with wax of one color, but this difference will be quickly erased. With due concentration it is relatively easy to apply the wax layers step by step and not in just one application.

Just as we can study interaction of reflected rays of light, we can also study different surface structures. This knowledge is particularly important because a carefully structured surface and its microgeography play an important role with regard to integration of the restoration in the patient's mouth.

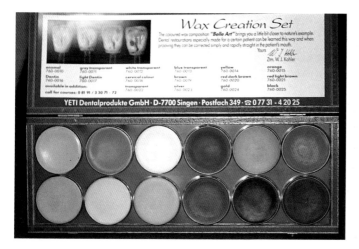
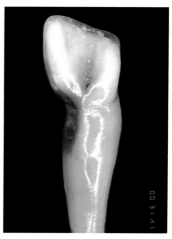

Figs 3-3 and 3-4 Using colored wax enables us to reproduce the shades of natural teeth and overcome the lack of perception by adding a three-dimensional aspect, ie, volume.

Psychological Advantages for Better Communication

Use of colored wax models ensures improved communication between dental laboratory, dentist, and patient. There is nothing worse than having to refabricate a restoration because of errors in shape, color, and other characteristics. In the case of repeated firings, liveliness and individuality are lost, as is motivation.

Under such difficulties it is more important to thoroughly study shape and characteristics using colored wax before ceramic work takes place (Figs 3-6 to 3-9).

Try-ins with provisional restorations – all made of colored wax – are of great psychological significance. They give the patient an idea of what the final restoration will look like (Figs 3-10 and 3-11). In this try-in phase, modifications are still possible and can be easily done. This saves a lot of back and forth between the dentist and the laboratory. Studies of the wax model beforehand can provide a solid basis for the final restoration. The ceramist, having already solved prob-

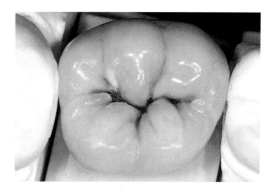

Fig 3-5 For the build-up of posterior teeth, colored wax is equally useful; three-dimensional occlusal concepts are easier to grasp.

lems of characterization and form, can fully concentrate on the process of fabrication and avoid time-consuming tries during the ceramic build-up process (Fig 3-12).

Colored wax provides a three-dimensional approach to dental anatomy and, at the same time, clearly shows the relation between

33

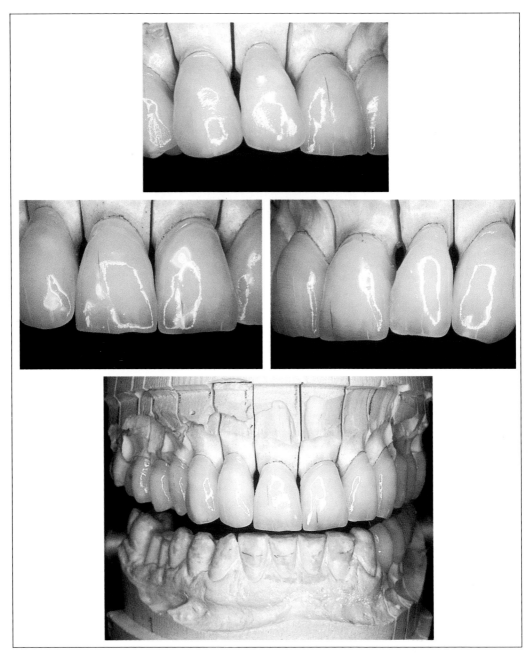

Figs 3-6 to 3-9 The use of colored wax supplies psychological advantages in communication between dental laboratory, dentist, and patient. Colored wax is essential to the study of tooth shape and characteristics.

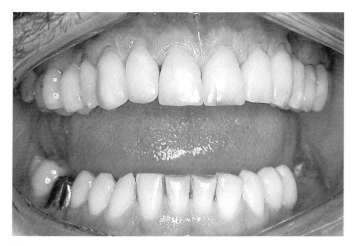 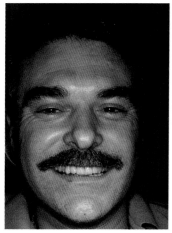

Figs 3-10 and 3-11 Try-ins of provisional restorations – all made of colored wax – with evaluation made while the restorations are placed inside the patient's mouth are of great psychological value. The patient then gets an idea of what the final restoration will look like.

Fig 3-12 Studies made beforehand with colored wax enable the ceramist to concentrate entirely on the ceramic during the build-up stage. Being free from thoughts about shape and characteristics, he can avoid awkward first attempts. Teeth 11, 12, 13, 21, 22, and 23 have been restored with metal ceramic crowns. (Clinical dentistry by Dr Daniel Gleyzolle, Avignon, France).

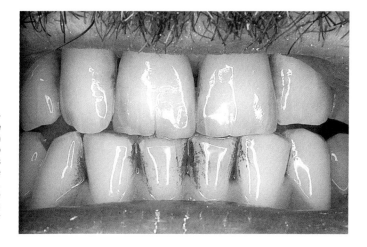

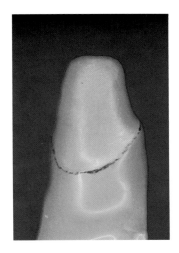
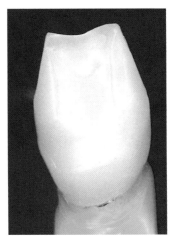

Fig 3-13 *(left)* Wax-up of a central maxillary incisor with colored wax. The first layer, being orange, produces a "warm" impression from underneath.

Fig 3-14 *(right)* For the wax-up the material is of the color of dentin.

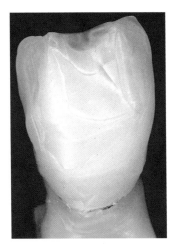
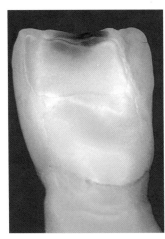

Figs 3-15 and 3-16 Orange-brown effects are added beneath the enamel layer in order to emphasize the infiltration of dentin. The proximal portions are built up using a transparent blue wax.

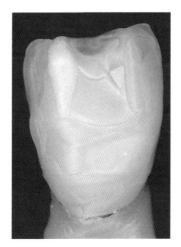 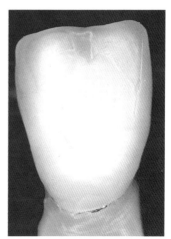

Fig 3-17 *(left)* Opalescent effects are applied.

Fig 3-18 *(right)* The tooth is wholly covered with a thin layer of transparent wax onto which an incisal wax is then applied.

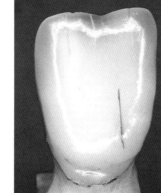 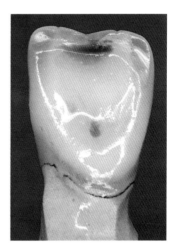

Fig 3-19 *(left)* Minor effects can be created with metal oxides.

Fig 3-20 *(right)* The crown wax-up is finished. The making of colored wax models can be coupled with incremental build-up of the porcelain. This is definitely an educational advantage, making the ceramic student's work somewhat easier.

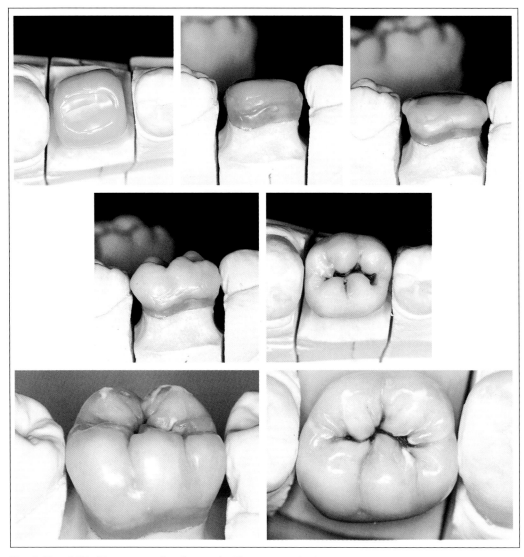

Figs 3-21 to 3-27 Wax-up procedure for a molar. The same method was used as described for the central incisor. The wax must be sufficiently hard to preserve the occlusal contacts.

color and shape (Figs 3-13 to 3-30). Aside from offering numerous psychological and educational advantages, this particular material and technique can also represent a source of satisfaction as well as motivation for the ceramist. A few reusable types of wax can form a comprehensive palette. If you cannot afford the time to do this by yourself, quality products are commercially available and can be purchased from dental suppliers.

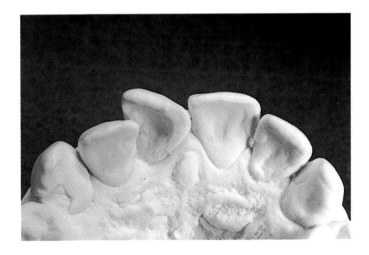

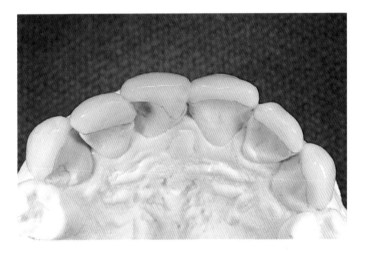

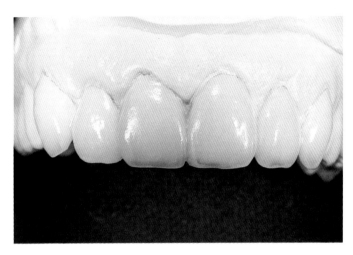

Figs 3-28 to 3-30 A study of the esthetics of veneers, produced with colored wax. The veneer has been slightly overcontoured in order to correct malalignment.

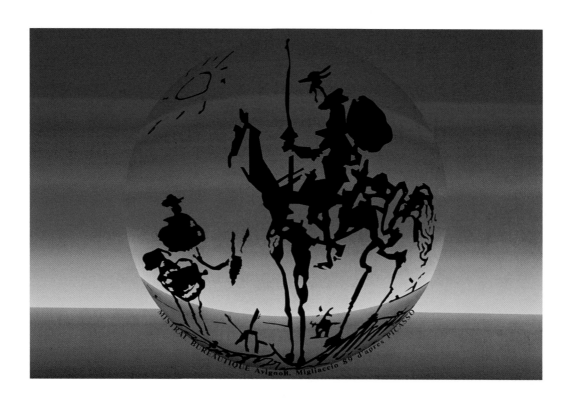

4   Color Selection

Determining the shading of teeth is an intricate process. Any shade selection made by the dentist is usually unreliable from our point of view, hence we do this step largely by ourselves. We think this is an adequate approach and should be pursued. It is equally as important for the ceramist to determine the color match as to check the placement of the restoration in the patient's mouth.

In the laboratory, shade selection is always made under the same source of light (eg, by Gamain, Paris).* Daylight is kept out using blinds. Always using the same source of light is most important. Daylight is too irregular; at daybreak the sky is reddish, in the evening and during the day it has a more blue hue. On top of that, you will find it impossible to have an identically colored sky every day.

Inside the laboratory, conditions for shade selection must always be identical. The walls and working station should be just one neutral color (gray) (Fig 4-1).

Moreover, the patient should not wear brightly colored clothes in close proximity to his or her teeth. Women should remove any lipstick because this, too, can negatively affect the result (Fig 4-2).

To select the suitable color, the entire range

* "Daylight" emanating from a ceiling lamp. Models 1865 and 1765, by Gamain (Paris). Color temperature: 6,500°K.

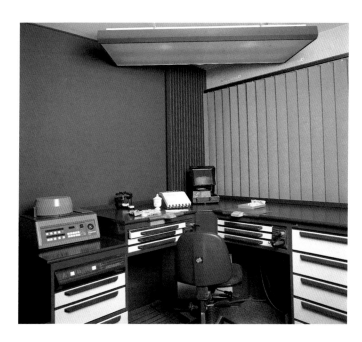

Fig 4-1   The color of a tooth should always be selected in an identical surrounding. Daylight should be kept out and a lamp like those made by Gamain (Paris) should be used.

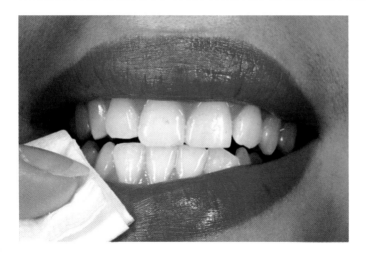

Fig 4-2 All colors deemed too bright can falsify the final result and must be removed: in this case, lipstick.

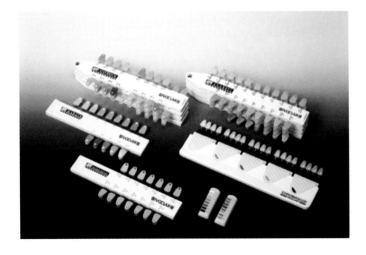

Fig 4-3 For color selection, all available shades of a ceramic shade guide system must be used.

of ceramic hues will be used (Fig 4-3). First we must choose the color group this tooth belongs to (yellow, yellowish-brown, etc) (Fig 4-4). Because prefabricated colors rarely match exactly those of a natural tooth you should settle for the closest one (Fig 4-5). It is therefore generally necessary to "create" a color (or "shade"). For that purpose the color must be broken down.

Breaking Down into Coats

First, the basic porcelain (opaque) must be chosen using a shade guide. The opaque porcelain is supposed to determine the color of the future restoration; metaphorically speaking, it is the "basis" of our canvas. The color of the opaque material should be more saturated than the color of the final restoration. You can hold a color sample next to the tooth in question if necessary. Even at this early stage you can control the final shade of

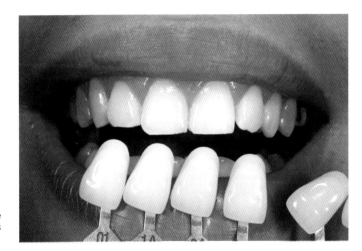

Fig 4-4 The first step is to determine the color group the tooth belongs with.

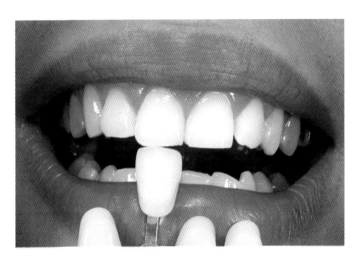

Fig 4-5 The color that is the closest match to the natural teeth will be selected. However, this rarely represents the right color.

a restoration by choosing a different opaque (Fig 4-6).

For instance, if the chosen color lacks brown, you can simply use an opaque porcelain that has more brown. After the opaque has been selected, the dentin porcelain is specified in the same way. Numerous kinds of dentin porcelains are available – quite original dentin colors as well as those of different color saturation (eg, dentin colors by Maverick). If there is no suitable dentin color, you can produce mixtures to obtain more subtle results. Dentin porcelain gained that way is then fired

to create a small custom shade guide for instant checks.

The selected dentin color should always be slightly more saturated because the build-up procedure progresses from saturated hues to less-saturated ones, and a nonsaturated dentin always overlies the dentin porcelain. If you do not use a saturated color as the first coat, the final color of the restored tooth will inevitably be too light (Fig 4-7).

For teeth with transparent incisal edges, the transparent porcelain must be selected accurately (Fig 4-8). A comprehensive palette

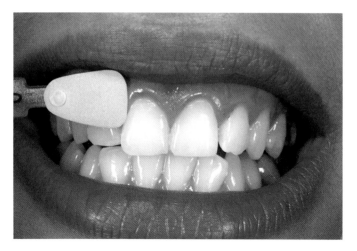

Fig 4-6 If the color the shade guide offers does not accurately match that of the natural tooth, we have to proceed by dividing the tooth's surface into different regions regarding color. The opaque basic color should be selected next. In this case the opaque matches only the cervical region. The color of the opaque must always be more saturated than that of the completed restoration.

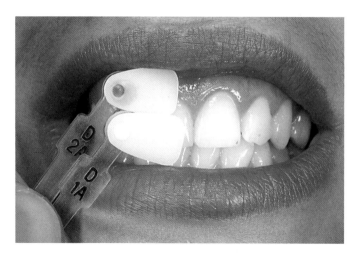

Fig 4-7 Selection of the dentin color. Frequently it will be necessary to use more than one color.

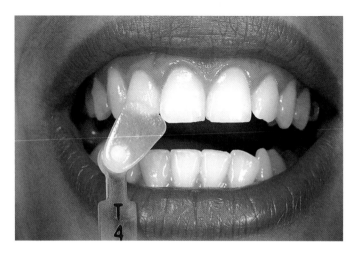

Fig 4-8 Selection of transparent and translucent porcelain. The transparent porcelain is barely visible.

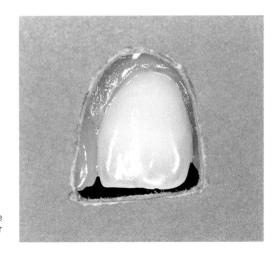

Fig 4-9   A "blinder" of neutral gray is used to separate the tooth from its surrounding, hence no nearby color can interfere with our judgment.

of transparent and translucent material should be used. Currently there is not only a range of gray hues available; instead, we are looking at a number of nine transparent and translucent materials, all of them moderately colored. Registration of all minor effects of a tooth's incisal edge must be perfect. The incisal third of anterior teeth is the most complex and difficult part to reconstruct. All colors are subtly nuanced and distributed. Here again Maverick's unsaturated dentin porcelains are of great help.

When selecting the color for anterior teeth, we use a small "blinder." This is a piece of neutral gray cardboard that has a cut-out in the centers about the size of a maxillary or mandibular central incisor. This blinder is held in front of the tooth to be restored, allowing us to observe only that tooth without being distracted by adjacent soft tissues or teeth (Fig 4-9).

Lastly, we select the matching incisal porcelain, of which often several are used (Fig 4-10). After the basic, dentin, and incisal porcelains have been selected, all effects and nuances are evaluated. Note that all indicators should be marked (Figs 4-11 and 4-12). We prefer to work with intense colors of a soft dentin rather than metal oxides because the latter are hard to handle and

quantify. Color selection is done not only for the labial surface but also for the lingual surface (Fig 4-13).

At times we must take color brilliance of teeth into consideration. In order to reduce the luminosity, a more gray opaque can be chosen and a transparent gray used as a last coat. This diminishes color brilliance (see chapter 5: "The Three-Dimensional Shade Guide and Changing Luminosity of Colors").

Having determined all parameters of color, we must never forget to record the surface structure of teeth that are to be restored. For this purpose the surface is cleaned with a paper tissue to remove saliva (Fig 4-14). Then characteristics in structure and the degree of surface luster are registered (see chapter 19: "Analysis of the Surface Structure – Polishing").

The search for and final selection of a specific color can prove most difficult, especially if that color must be custom mixed. With regard to efficiency, we regard the technique described here as one of the best, or at least as being practical and reasonable. However, as with any method, there is a subjective component to the selection of color, and it strongly demands profound knowledge about the build-up of ceramic.

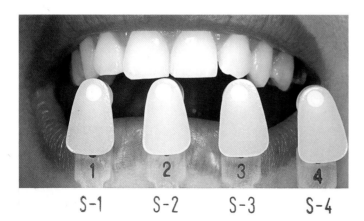

S-1   S-2   S-3   S-4

Fig 4-10 The incisal porcelain is determined. A single specimen rarely suffices.

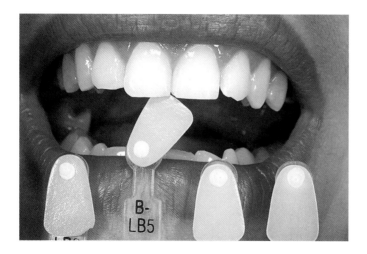

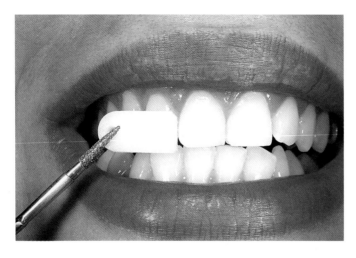

Figs 4-11 and 4-12 Every effect the tooth shows must be considered. *(above)* Color selection for the incisal edge ("halo effect"). *(left)* Selection of opalescent regions.

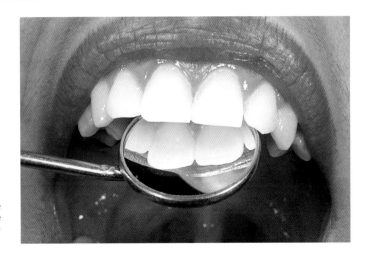

Fig 4-13 Determination for the lingual surface. From this angle the teeth show other interesting characteristics.

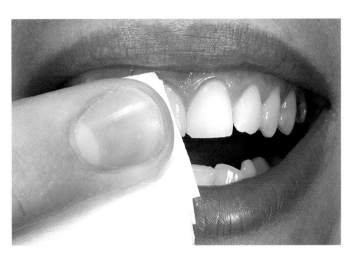

Fig 4-14 Saliva must be removed to allow unrestricted observation of the tooth surface, its texture, and the degree of luster.

5   The Three-Dimensional Shade Guide and Changing Luminosity of Colors

When selecting tooth colors, frequently it is the color brilliance that proves difficult to evaluate and register. The most difficult part is therefore not selecting the correct hue; regarding the degree of saturation it is rather simple. But with color brilliance, the amount of gray components a color contains makes it much more complicated. None of the known systems of shade guides makes it any easier to choose between several degrees of luminosity of one specific color.

Communication between the dentist and the dental technician concerning color selection is often imprecise. The reason is unsuitable shade guides and, in particular, a complete lack of information on color brilliance, which is hard to judge.

It should be possible nowadays to improve brilliance control on the existing shade guides.

When the color brilliance of a tooth is too bright although the saturation and basic color are correct, there are two ways to remedy the situation:

The first method (which I regard as unsatisfactory) involves applying a coat of gray metal oxide to the surface during the glaze bake; it is possible to reduce the brilliance when a combined gray is used. This method has one major drawback, however. There is no way to mechanically polish the ceramic surface without also removing the oxides.

The second method involves applying a very thin coat of gray transparent porcelain. This coat does not influence the color or its saturation but merely corrects the degree of luminosity. Afterwards it is possible to polish the ceramic.

This method is frequently used to correct color brilliance. Therefore, we have added three facets of brilliance to the shade guide (ie, shade guide for study purposes) (Fig 5-1). These facets correspond to three ceramic powders of translucent gray:
1. Light gray: 2 parts T4 + 1 part gray ID8,
2. Grayer: 1 part T4 + 2 parts gray ID8,
3. Grayest: pure ID8.

These three facets are placed on the ceramic facets of the shade guide and thus modify their luminosity (Fig 5-2). If we do not find a proper correspondent in brilliance for the tooth to be restored despite a suitable opaque and good color saturation, a facet is placed against the ceramic teeth to obtain a distinct nuance. This will correct the color brilliance. Later we can check inside the patient's mouth whether our correction corresponds with the color brilliance of the natural teeth. If this is not the case we repeat the procedure with the two other, grayer facets. Once the three dimensions of color have been determined it is easy to record the appropriate color-reference (eg, color brilliance 1, 2, or 3).

In the laboratory when fabricating a ceramic restoration we use the build-up technique; except that when the last layer is to be applied we use a translucent gray. This does not alter the basic color or saturation, it merely influences the brilliance (Fig 5-3).

For accurate determination of color brilliance of a natural tooth, this method is simple and feasible. The process of selecting colors

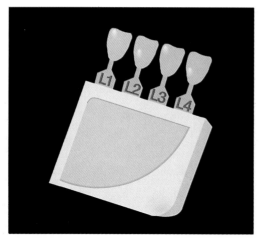

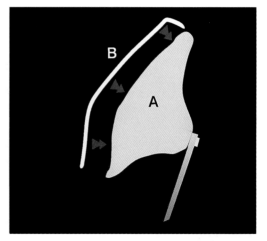

Fig 5-1 A custom shade guide composed of several facets of different luminosity. This shade guide enables the determination of the gray portion of a tooth. It is a completion of the commercially available shade guide systems and is the first guide to include the three-dimensional aspect. The scale ranges from the lightest to the grayest nuance (L1, L2, L3, L4).

Fig 5-2 Each luminosity facet (B) can be clamped to a commercial shade guide (A). The facets influence and change the brilliance of a tooth. For each of the four degrees of luminosity a range of four different porcelains is provided. These porcelains are incrementally applied during build-up of a tooth to consequently obtain the desired color brilliance.

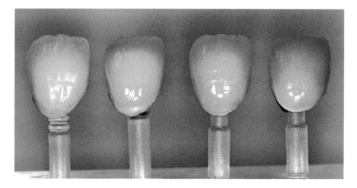

Fig 5-3 These four porcelain teeth are identical in terms of hue and saturation. They are distinguished only by their brilliance. On the far left is the tooth with the highest luminosity and on the far right is the tooth with the highest amount of gray. Clearly the color of teeth can be influenced by incremental application of porcelain mass containing more or less gray (L1, L2, or L3). It is possible to quantify a tooth's color brilliance using facets of different degrees of luminosity.

and communicating the result from dentist to dental technician is thereby improved; moreover, the investment is minimal – three additional powder jugs. It would be even more convenient to have three gray plastic facets that can be adapted perfectly and contrast distinctly with the nuances of the shade guide.

For the future it will be important that manufacturers provide systems of shade guides with nuances that represent all three brilliance dimensions in order to make dentist – technician communication easier. And we propose that our nuanced luminosity system is on the right path!

6 Instruments

Technicians who work with dental ceramics must have profound knowledge of the ceramic material as well as of tooth morphology, occlusion, and color. Last but not least, they must also have the ability to observe – plus have an artistic streak. All of the above, though, will not suffice without appropriate instruments and accurate methods chosen for every single step. Because of organizational and simplifying reasons we prefer to work with a minimum of instruments; hence repeated manipulations are simplified and will not distract the ceramist's concentration.

Modeling brush. The modeling brush we use is of medium size, big enough to function as a reservoir for water in order to maintain a constant degree of humidity while modeling. It is made of selected, pure hair of a marten's fur, thus it has great density and a very sharp point similar to that of a stinger. Using the same brush we can, for purposes of rapid modeling, remove surplus ceramic material and wipe it off on a paper napkin, as well as form even the most difficult incisal edges incrementally, thanks to its flame shape. With its very sharp point we can recontour the occlusal fissures for the second firing. The high-quality marten's hair provides the brush with a variable geometry so we can exclusively use only this one modeling brush (by Prodentax, Lyon, France). However, these

Fig 6-2 The very sharp yet dense point of this brush can serve as an aid for shaping occlusal surfaces and recontouring fissures.

Fig 6-1 Modeling brush: this brush is foldable and a removable cap ensures that moisture can be maintained for several hours. Its original flame-shape and density will also be preserved.

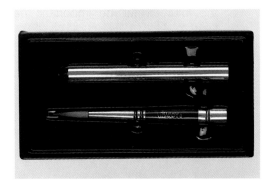

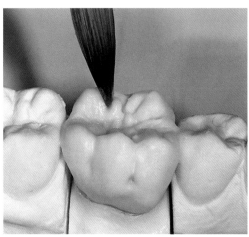

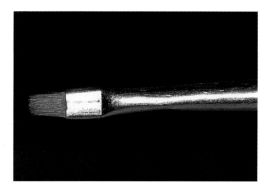

Fig 6-3 The brush for enamel cracks has a flat point not unlike a chisel edge.

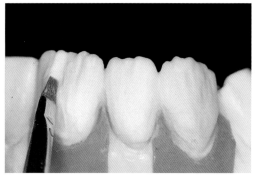

Fig 6-4 This brush can be used to mimic cracks on stress-bearing areas of the tooth. Because of its chisel-like point, a very defined area can be stained.

characteristics will be rapidly lost if the brush is not protected. Therefore, a removable cap must be used to preserve moisture for several hours or even until the next day. The original flame shape and density of the brush's hair will also be preserved in this way (Figs 6-1 and 6-2).

Brush for enamel cracks. This brush is quite small (no. 2), flat, fine, and has a square point. It, too, is made of choice marten's hair. It is especially designed for lateral segmentation and is used to create the illusion of enamel cracks. The flat shape obviously predestined the brush for that purpose. It is also possible to apply staining colors in order to mimic cracks on stress-bearing segments. A brush with a pointed tip would only permit the application of fine streaks of color. The square-pointed brush, on the contrary, permits small, colored patches, which give natural cracks the appearance of depth (Figs 6-3 and 6-4).

Whipping brush. This brush is the thickest of all. Its hair is not marten's hair but is horse's hair instead. It is very soft, not at all stiff. It can be used after finalization of the ceramic build-up to produce a well-rounded shape. Moreover, it can impart to the entire restoration a

certain fragility because of its own softness. The tool is used to brush the occlusal surfaces in the direction of the fissures (Fig 6-5), and it is of great help in producing ceramic shoulders, where the brush is worked in an incisocervical direction.

"Painting" brush. This brush is rarely used and is not considered appropriate for the amateur, who tends to overdo the application of staining colors. It is extremely fine (no. 00) and made of marten's hair. The main function of this brush is to apply staining colors, which are used to mimic all sorts of discolorations natural teeth exhibit: partially or completely stained fissures or interproximal spaces, and discolorations of concave areas of the tooth. This brush also must be very dense, in order to meet all these conditions.

Opaque "glass stick". This is surely the cheapest of all instruments and is available in any pharmacy because one can use an ordinary medical ampule. The very end of the ampule should be smooth and rounded and, if possible, slightly bent. Using this device it is possible to apply opaque porcelain without any water. The method is quick and leads to very even and smooth surfaces (Fig 6-6).

Multifunctional separating spatula. This

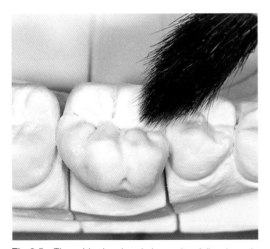

Fig 6-5 The whipping brush is made of fine horse's hair. It is useful for fabricating porcelain margins and cleaning occlusal surfaces; the stroke must always be in direction of the fissures.

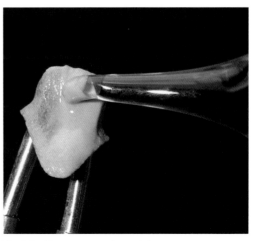

Fig 6-6 The opaque glass stick.

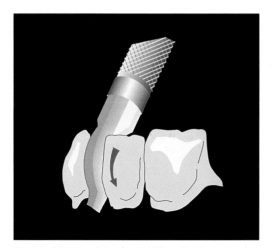

Fig 6-7 The semicircular multifunctional separating spatula is used during the build-up process on fixed partial dentures and pontics.

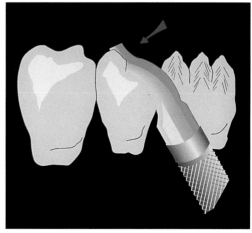

Fig 6-8 The straight and cutting edge of this two-sided instrument helps to cut off fine tips of excess porcelain.

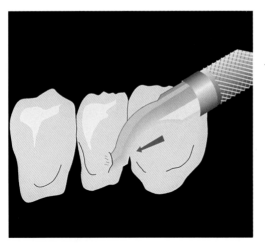

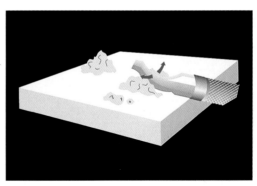

Fig 6-10 Because of its flexible blade, the multifunctional spatula works well for mixing porcelain or metal oxides.

Fig 6-9 The same instrument is used here to erode the porcelain mass; its fine, flat tip is particularly helpful in pressure-packing the porcelain particles during correction and second firing.

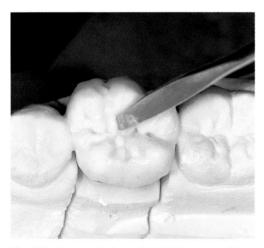

Fig 6-11 The spatula is used to fabricate natural-looking fissures. All fissures are produced with this instrument; we do not advocate use of rotary instruments. The spatula should be flat, smooth, and slightly bent at the rounded tip, to adapt well to the shape of cusps.

instrument can be used in many ways. We modified a flexible razor blade. Its original shape has many functions: to separate the pontics of a metal ceramic bridge (Fig 6-7), cut off excess ceramic tips (Fig 6-8), erode the ceramic or, for the second bake of a ceramic fixed partial denture, to condense the correction porcelain (Fig 6-9). This spatula can also be used for mixing the ceramic (Fig 6-10).

Spatula to produce natural-looking fissures. This instrument is indispensable for creating natural-looking occlusal surfaces. Because fissures never run in straight lines we use this spatula and not a rotary instrument to work with untreated dental porcelain. The spatula should be flat, smooth, and slightly bent at the rounded tip, to adapt well to the shape of cusps (Fig 6-11).

Mixing spatula. This spatula should be made of plastic, to avoid any contact of the mixing slab – which is consistently kept moist – and metal. When mixing, it is very important not to trap any air in the porcelain. The ceramist should observe carefully that the porcelain exhibits a soft and workable consistency.

Diamond-tip tweezers. These two tweezers

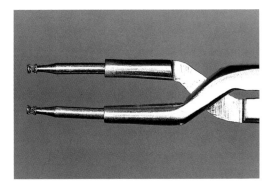

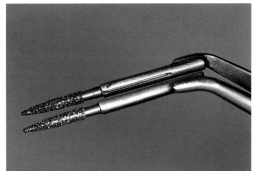

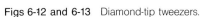

Figs 6-12 and 6-13 Diamond-tip tweezers.

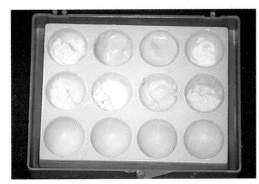

Fig 6-14 The constant humidity box maintains a certain degree of moisture that is essential for dental porcelain processing.

are essential for manipulating ceramic material that must not be touched with bare fingers. They make transport and placement on the heat-resistant plate easier during surface characterization (Figs 6-12 and 6-13).

Constant humidity box. In order to obtain pleasing results, the ceramist must follow one simple rule: dental porcelain always has to be processed under a constant degree of humidity, which provides the material with plasticity that is extremely helpful for modeling. It is not possible to obtain a moist powder of good quality on a glass slab. Therefore, we use a glass slab in a box of constant humidity (Fig 6-14). There is a reservoir of distilled water underneath the slab that will maintain the same degree of humidity even for a few days. Economical aspects ought not to be neglected when working with ceramic powder.

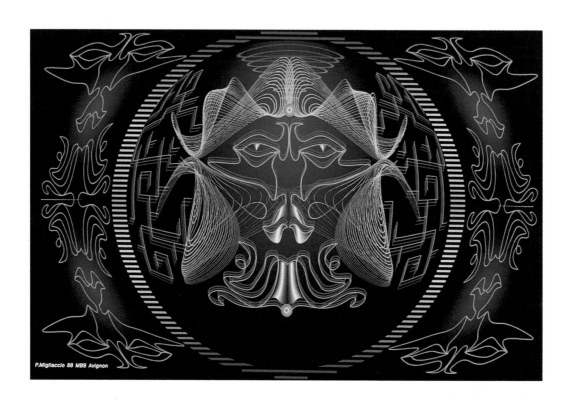

7 Basic (Opaque) Porcelains

The application of basic porcelain may seem of subordinate importance for the ceramist's work. However, it is a difficult and serious step. From the ceramist's viewpoint the opaque should represent the final shade of a tooth. This is the layer of highest saturation and will appear to be more or less intense depending on the thickness of the ensuing coats of ceramic material. The main function of the basic porcelain is to mask the metal substructure. But light penetrating the ceramic and being reflected by the metal causes undesirable effects, in particular because of the gray reflection of metal oxides. The thickness of application determines the quality of the opaque porcelain layer. Hence, to avoid all gray reflections on cervical or buccal surfaces we use covering gold; only a very thin layer of opaque material will then be necessary.

Application of Opaque Porcelains

Opaque "wash". T!he opaque wash is not supposed to fully mask the metal substructure with just one single layer; rather, it establishes a link between the metal substructure and the so-called covering gold (Fig 7-1). Its hue is inconspicuous, possibly neutral to avoid any unwanted influence from the layers underneath. We use the glass stick for distribution of the wash. It is necessary to moisten the metal surface gently in order to facilitate further wetting. The application must be done rapidly to prevent the thin coat from drying too soon. The opaque wash is slightly condensed at the same time.

Covering gold coat. In order to rule out any gray reflections caused by the opaque, a covering gold coat is used. It is commercially available as a paste (Keradec by Wieland, Düsseldorf, Germany). The kit contains a liquid with which the paste is thinned to creamy consistency. The material can then be easily applied to the entire surface of the substructure with a small brush. It is not advisable to apply covering gold only on the cervical region. Even with sufficient thickness of the ceramic layer, the substructure's gray reflections will influence the color. According to the manufacturers, this gold coat will only be a negligible 10 to 15 µm thick. After the application, the coping is dried in the furnace for 6 minutes. The initial temperature of 600°C should be raised at a rate of 60°C per minute to a final 820°C. After firing, the covering gold should have a matte finish; it should not shine because this would provoke too much reflection (Fig 7-2). By using covering gold the cervical edges show a yellowish-gold appearance instead of an unpleasant gray tinge from the metal substructure.

Application of dentin porcelain. This opaque component represents the color that was specified. It should mask the covering gold. If its layer shows some irregularities in thickness, even the thinnest areas will cause no disadvantage because the coat is completely underlayed by the covering gold's yellow color. The opaque should be of creamy consistency; when applied with a glass stick, the opaque can be thinly distributed. Prior to the application, the metal substructure must be slightly moistened in order to facilitate further wetting.

The opaque is to be applied from top to bottom, ie, from occlusal/incisal to cervical

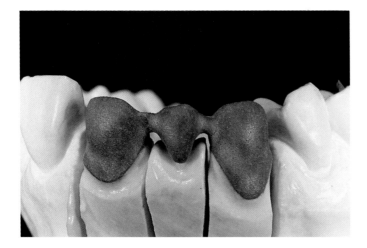

Fig 7-1 Opaque wash covering the substructure after firing. The opaque wash should not mask the metal substructure fully with just one single layer; rather it should establish a link between the metal substructure and the so-called covering gold.

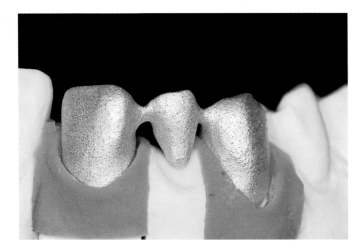

Fig 7-2 The covering gold should not shine after firing, because this would produce too much reflection; it should have a matte finish.

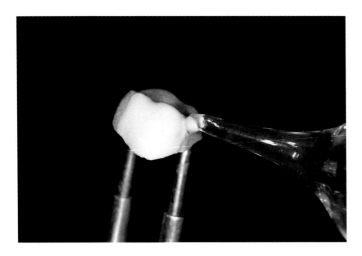

Fig 7-3 Opaque application using a glass rod. The tip of a medical ampule is handy for this purpose. The material is applied from top to bottom; distinct transitions should be covered last.

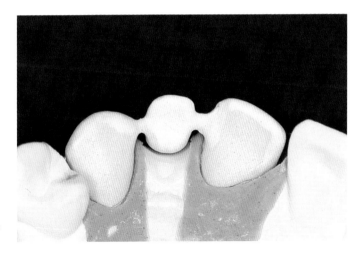

Fig 7-4 After firing the opaque should have an eggshell appearance.

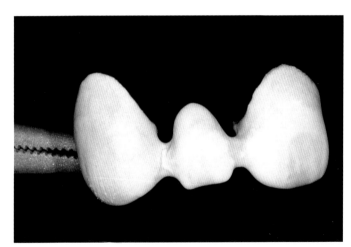

Fig 7-5 The colored opaque material. The coloration may be diffuse or show distinct boundaries, according to the shade guide.

surfaces; the occlusal surfaces and distinct transitions should be covered last (Fig 7-3). The material is condensed with a few light and gentle taps. After firing, the opaque should have an eggshell appearance. Above all it should not shine, because that would create too strong a reflection and would thus impair the final result (Fig 7-4).

Modifying the opaque. Generally, the opaque is not colored too conspicuously. In most cases we prefer to use intense dentin porcelain to reproduce all internal shades. However, this is only possible when the ce-

ramic restoration is 1 or 2 mm thick. If the restoration is thinner, color and its characteristic features must be considered during the opaque application. Selecting the right hue for the basic porcelain is of major importance; this may be achieved either by use of intense opaque or with the application of metal oxides, thus staining the opaque layer. The opaque must be colored during application, which may look as blurred as a photograph of the earth taken from space or show distinct junctions according to the shade guide (Fig 7-5). The opaque should

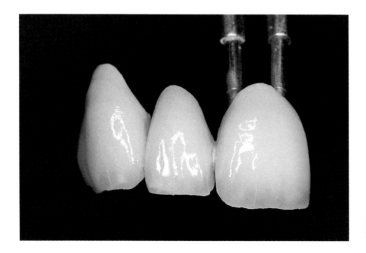

Fig 7-6 The completed fixed partial denture.

be condensed with a few gentle taps with the spatula. This gentle condensation will draw the particles together; however, vibration should be avoided because it could shift the layers and force them into concavities. The basic porcelains are allowed to dry well before they are fired. A drying time of 5 minutes is scheduled; the temperature is raised at a rate of 80°C per minute, a little quicker than firing of the dentin porcelain (60°C per minute) (Fig 7-6).

Coloring the opaque makes it possible to master even difficult situations, such as underreduction and consequently lack of thickness. This technique can trick the eye because it creates the appearance of volume and depth. However, it must not be used excessively for it may lead to results where reduction of luminosity is important and correction with adequate thickness of porcelain is no longer possible.

8   The Ceramic Shoulder

The ceramic shoulder represents considerable progress in our endeavor for better esthetics. Generally, we are tempted to use ceramic for restoration of the margin as often as possible, particularly with anterior teeth. Provided the technique is mastered well, no precision will be lost. In general, the labial portion of a restoration is produced with a ceramic shoulder, but the entire margin of the restoration can be fabricated in ceramic if the preparation permits. This requires a wide, full-shoulder formation. To obtain excellent precision, two firings will be necessary.

Prerequisites for a Ceramic Shoulder

In order to fabricate a ceramic shoulder, the preparation must be adequate. A wide, circumferential shoulder and an angle of 90° is propitious. For optimal esthetic results, it is desirable to have a restoration margin 1 mm thick (Fig 8-1).

Preparing the Die

Prior to the porcelain application, the cervical edges of the preparation must be marked with a wax crayon. Great care must be exercised not to soften the right-angled finish line of the prepared shoulder. This is essential for accurate marginal fit of the restoration. Denudation of the cervical margin means careful preservation of the area where the root portion of the die begins. The beginning

of the root portion will later be a guideline for the crown margin. It is useful to apply some hardening varnish to the die in order to secure the wax crayon marks and harden the well-defined cervical margin (ie, the shoulder edge). These marks as well as the shoulder edge are thus protected. This varnish works like a protective shield, preventing the die from absorbing the moisture of the subsequently applied porcelain. A cyano-varnish is used as hardener, but not before a first coat of gray and a second coat of gold die spacer have been applied.

First Shoulder Porcelain Bake

Before the porcelain is applied, the die must be treated with a separating wax pencil (Fig 8-2). The shoulder porcelain is mixed with liquid to a creamy consistency. Substructures for ceramic restorations should exhibit very gentle friction, and above all, no undercut should create an impediment. The porcelain is applied directly to the lower portion of the metal coping without touching the prepared portion of the die (Fig 8-3). We do not pack by condensing but use a paper napkin to press the porcelain onto the shoulder. The napkin absorbs excess moisture and prevents the porcelain from adhering to the die (Fig 8-4). When the coping is removed there will be no excess ceramic at the edges. The die is separated again and the coping reseated. A very soft brush is used to shift the porcelain in the direction of the cervical finish line while it is

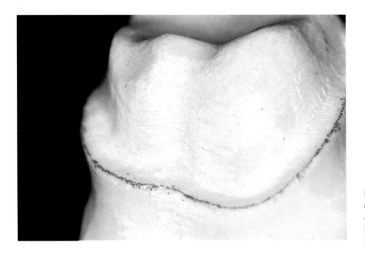

Fig 8-1 The required width of an esthetic porcelain shoulder is 1 mm at least. The preparation margin should be accurate and show a 90° angle all around.

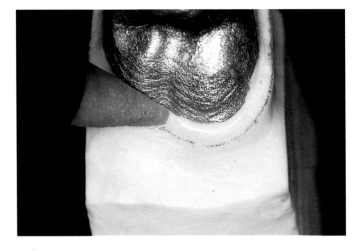

Fig 8-2 The shoulder is shown prior to the application of the porcelain and is separated with a wax pencil.

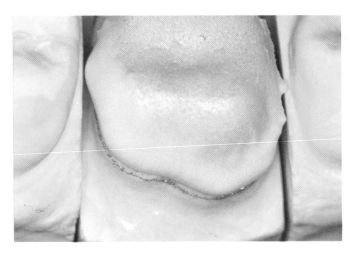

Fig 8-3 The porcelain is applied directly to the lower edge of the metal coping without touching the prepared portion of the die.

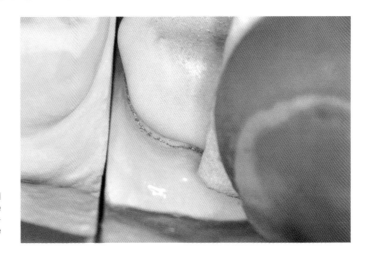

Fig 8-4 A paper napkin is used to press the porcelain onto the shoulder. The napkin absorbs excess moisture and prevents the porcelain from adhering to the die.

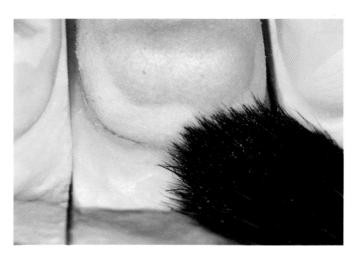

Fig 8-5 Using a soft brush of horse's hair, the porcelain is shifted in the direction of the cervical finish line while it is still moist.

still moist (Fig 8-5). All excess material is carefully removed using the blade of a scalpel. The coping is lifted off the die, and the marginal fit of the porcelain will exhibit a clean edge and be accurate. Now the first bake can be performed.

Second Shoulder Porcelain Bake

After the firing and before the coping is reseated on the die, a fine-grit diamond is used to free the internal surface of small porcelain nodules that may cause problems when reseating. This initial check can disclose a small opening caused by firing shrinkage, but the main reason for that marginal deficiency is that we omitted to condense the porcelain slurry. In order to fill in that opening, a mix of moist shoulder powder and special glazing liquid is prepared. This considerably thicker liquid prevents the thin corrective material from drying prematurely. The same liquid is used to lightly cover the edge of the baked ceramic to facilitate further wetting (Fig 8-6). A small bulge of shoulder

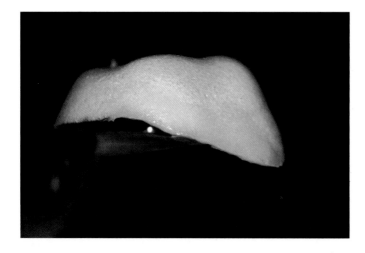

Fig 8-6 After the first bake a correction porcelain is applied with a spatula. In order to facilitate further wetting, glazing liquid is lightly applied to the edge of the ceramic.

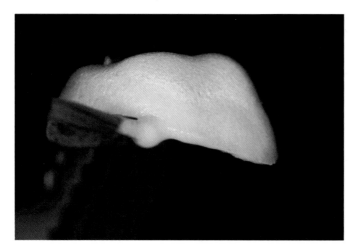

Fig 8-7 A small bulge of shoulder porcelain mixed with some glazing liquid is applied to this edge.

porcelain is later applied to this area (Fig 8-7). The coping is reseated on the die by exerting gentle pressure after the separating pencil has been carefully used once more (Fig 8-8). This time, the material is lightly condensed and excess moisture is absorbed with a paper tissue to ensure proper adaptation of the coping.

Again, we lift the coping off the die, treat the die with the separating wax pencil, reseat the coping, and ensure a perfect marginal fit while stroking gently with a flexible brush in an occlusocervical direction. Finally, the cop-

ing is removed in order to proceed to the second bake. The firing is done according to the usual program. The more viscous liquid prevents the thin corrective porcelain from drying out or crumbling away.

After the second porcelain bake, the formation of the ceramic shoulder is virtually finished (Fig 8-9). Now the full crown contour can be established. Only when the restoration has been completed (ie, after the glaze bake) will the correction firing be done. For this purpose a mix of shoulder porcelain and 20% to 30% glazing powder (low-fusing por-

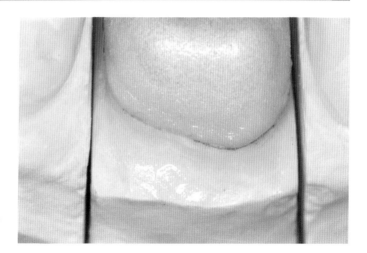

Fig 8-8 The unfinished restoration is reseated on the die while exerting slight pressure.

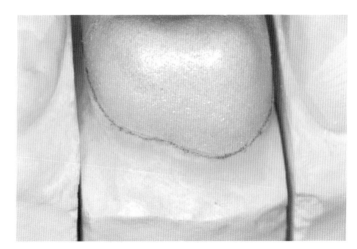

Fig 8-9 After the second porcelain bake, the ceramic shoulder is virtually finished. Now the full crown contour can be established. Only when the restoration has been completed (ie, after the glaze bake) will the correction firing be done.

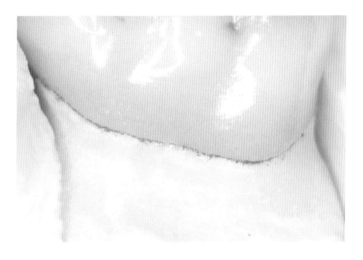

Fig 8-10 Finally, the ceramic margin is polished with a carborundum polisher and the marginal fit is inspected.

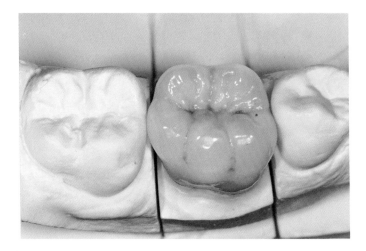

Fig 8-11 The completed restoration after polishing.

celain) is used. This reduces the fusion temperature of the corrective porcelain. Possible minor inaccuracies are generally corrected in this fashion. After firing, the ceramic margin can be finished with an abrasive stone; the marginal fit is then checked (Fig 8-10).

The fabrication of a ceramic shoulder is not an easy task. Therefore, we advise a method that is precise as well as efficient and easy to adopt. Essential prerequisites for success are well-defined and clean, right-angled finish lines (Fig 8-11).

9 Artificial Gingiva

In general, ceramists in commercial laboratories work isolated from dentist and patient. Dental technology and dentistry are different but complementary professions; the best restorations originate from well-balanced teamwork between the two. Most of the dental laboratories, including ours, are located some distance away from their dentist customers. Communication is one of many elements that contribute to success. Therefore, any technique that improves communication in daily practice is helpful.

Artificial gingiva is also an element we cannot do without in daily laboratory procedures. We have used this technique for many years now, and it is difficult to imagine dentistry without it. Artificial gingiva has been particularly useful with anterior teeth, where poor design of interproximal space is the major cause of poor esthetics.

Using the artificial gingiva, it is possible to design interproximal areas with reduced compression on adjacent soft tissues and improved access for interproximal brushes for the periodontally compromised patient.

The junction from the tooth's hard tissue to the surrounding gingival soft tissues and the faciocervical contour must be clearly visible. The contour of the cervical third can obviously be derived from the morphology of the periodontal vicinity (Fig 9-1).

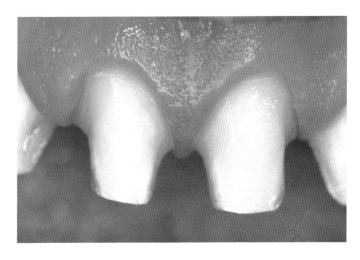

Fig 9-1 How do we visualize the gingiva when the teeth have been prepared for crown restorations? It is almost impossible to assess the topography of the sulcus and the risk of gingival compression without using artificial gingiva. (Tooth preparation by Dr Luc Portalier.)

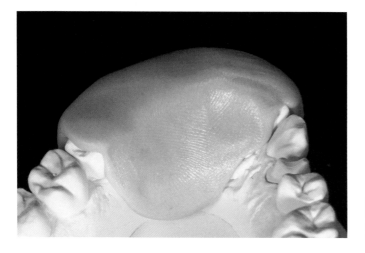

Fig 9-2 An impression is made of the prepared teeth and the adjacent soft tissue using a highly viscous silicone compound.

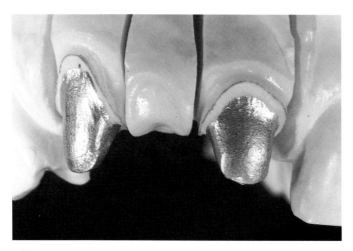

Fig 9-3 The dies are separated and ground to the desired shape.

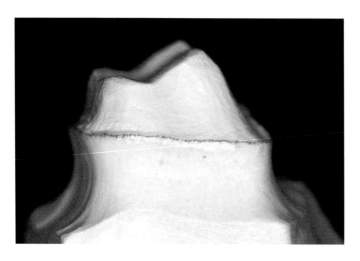

Fig 9-4 The die has been prepared and the finishing line is denuded before the artificial gingiva is fabricated.

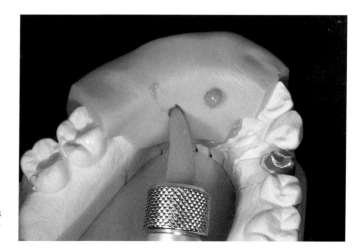

Fig 9-5 A low-viscosity silicone is injected with a syringe (ESPE-Premier) into the prepared openings.

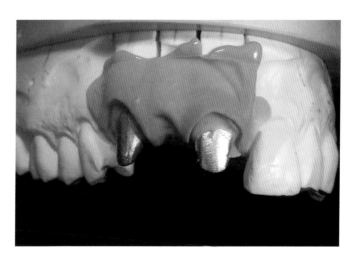

Fig 9-6 The artificial gingiva after the excess silicone has been removed and the index has been lifted off the cast.

Fabrication of Removable Artificial Gingiva

First an index of the unprepared cast is made using a high-viscosity silicone compound (Fig 9-2). The soft tissues must be accurately duplicated. Then the cast is separated, and the die is trimmed to show the finish line (Fig 9-3); a 4-mm round tungsten grinder is used. This grinder helps to provide sufficient space beneath the cervical margin for the silicone (Fig 9-4). The lingual wall of the index is perforated several times to provide for

canals that can be used to inject a low-viscosity silicone compound. After the index is repositioned on the working cast, the compound is injected with an impression syringe to fill the void (Fig 9-5). The compound sets, the soft compound excess is cut off, and the index is lifted off the working cast (Fig 9-6). The gingiva is duplicated by the compound representing the impression. The artificial gingiva is removed and excess silicone is cut off using a pointed tungsten grinder or a pair of scissors (Figs 9-7 and 9-8). The entire procedure takes only a few minutes. The fabri-

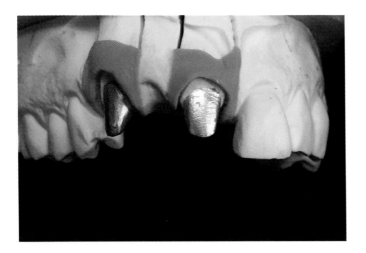

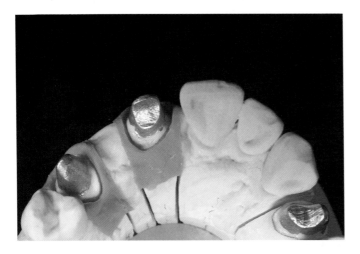

Figs 9-7 and 9-8 All excess silicone has been removed and the artificial gingiva is trimmed.

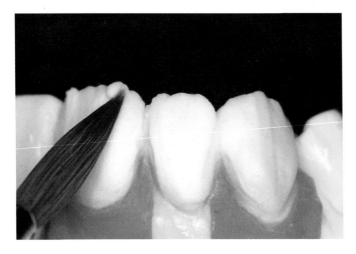

Fig 9-9 The artificial gingiva is very helpful during the porcelain build-up stage; it facilitates a quick assessment of form and cervical contour and enables better adaptation of crown margins to the adjacent tissues.

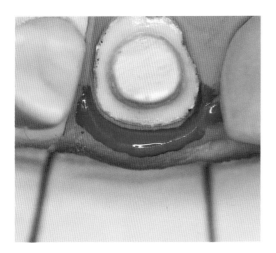

Fig 9-10 An elastomeric detection paste is used to identify regions of undesirable compression of the periodontium.

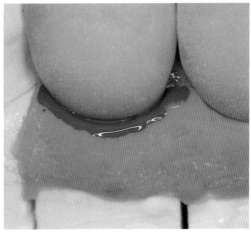

Fig 9-11 The crown is seated on the die; if any compression is present, it will bounce back.

cated gingiva is a considerable aid for defining the periodontal surrounding and its relation to esthetics (Figs 9-9 to 9-12). The duplication of the soft tissues will differ from the natural gingiva in volume by one tenth of a millimeter due to shrinkage of the impression, but this is a negligible discrepancy in relation to the benefit of the procedure. The only risk is minor compression, which can be compensated for by grinding back the porcelain during a try-in of the unfinished restoration.

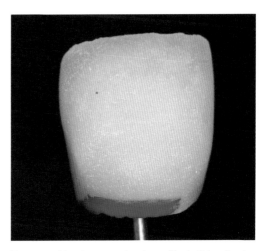

Fig 9-12 After the crown has been lifted off the die, the regions of compression are clearly marked and can be eliminated.

10 Processing and Natural Layering of Metal Ceramic

Every committed dental technician has studied sections of natural teeth in the attempt to mimic their internal structures. The author is one of those who collect cross sections and photographs in order to study nature as closely as possible. Sectioned teeth best show the main characteristics that are significant for the fabrication of restorations in dental porcelain, no matter if metal ceramic or all-ceramic.

From the sectioned natural teeth in Figs 10-1 to 10-4 the following conclusions can be drawn: all teeth exhibit a distinct color saturation in their center that decreases toward the periphery. The cross sections of ceramic teeth in Figs 10-5 and 10-6 show a central portion of high saturation representing the pulp; a variety of dentin porcelain was used, highly saturated in the center and less saturated toward the periphery, all covered by several layers of transparent and incisal porcelains.

There is a transparent zone beneath the enamel that apparently facilitates the circulation of light inside the tooth. This is a contradiction to the traditional way of modeling in dental ceramics. It is common practice to apply the transparent porcelain onto the incisal surface. This results in well-shaped restorations seated on the working cast, but they do not look natural. In general, the core of the internal structure is sectioned by the dark background of the oral cavity behind.

In Figs 10-5 and 10-6 the transparent layer is quite discernible because it underlies the enamel porcelain. It conveys light, somewhat like a fiberoptic cable. Figure 10-5 clearly depicts the formation of different layers at the periphery as well as the layer of incisal por-

celain, which overlies the transparent material. The purpose behind studying these teeth is to improve imitation of natural teeth (Figs 10-7 and 10-8). However, these cross-sectioned teeth are merely part of our studies and become significant only when the previous observations can be applied in daily laboratory procedures. We therefore produced a cross-sectioned metal ceramic crown (Figs 10-9 and 10-10) fabricated with different kinds of dentin porcelain, going from the most saturated to the most opaque, where the opaque determines the color of the porcelain build-up. The dentin porcelain was incrementally layered, thus decreasing the saturation: altogether three kinds of dentin porcelains, and the enamel porcelain superimposed on the transparent porcelain. This cross section of a metal ceramic crown is schematic but nicely illustrates that method.

We have always fabricated our restorations with the incremental build-up and lateral segmentation techniques. These two methods are complementary and lead to very satisfying results (Figs 10-11 and 10-12). However, we do not use condensation (ie, the packing of the porcelain particles) to obtain higher density because all effects, layers, and segmentations disappear and form just one mix after condensation.

From basic knowledge of painting and color theory, we know that the three primary colors, if mixed in the correct quantities, yield black. This fact applies to painting as well as dental porcelain, where gray is the result if too many colors are mixed. Therefore, the application of different porcelains adjacent to each other (lateral segmentation technique) or layers of porcelain (layering technique) is

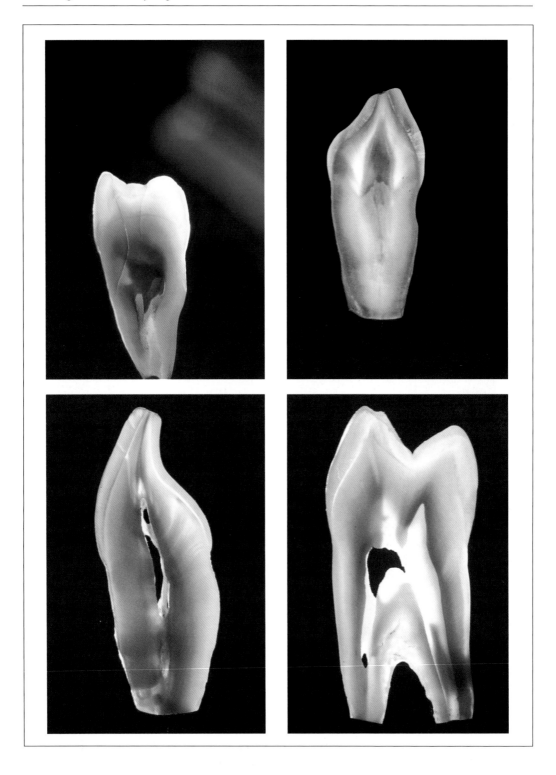

Figs 10-1 to 10-4 Two facts can be observed in these photographs of vertical cross sections of natural teeth. The color is saturated in the center and becomes lighter at the margins. Furthermore, the zone of transparency is always located beneath the enamel layer. The light circulates beneath the enamel, a phenomenon that is particularly distinct in Figs 10-3 and 10-4.

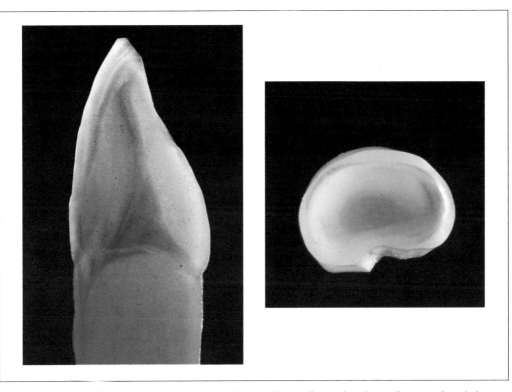

Figs 10-5 and 10-6 These all-ceramic teeth were fabricated according to the observations mentioned above on natural teeth: *(1)* The teeth have been fabricated according to the build-up technique, ie, from saturated color in the center to less saturated color at the periphery, and *(2)* the transparent material has been applied beneath a layer of incisal porcelain. Light can circulate just as it does within natural teeth. The highly saturated color in the center mimics the color of the pulp.

recommended in order to accomplish natural-looking rather than gray-appearing restorations, reminiscent of the impressionists who used to work their brushes in a stippling manner (see chapter 1, "Basic Terms of the Phenomenon of Color"). Condensed porcelain consequently means condensed particle distribution, thus resulting in a restoration of impaired translucent appearance.

Every ceramist and colorist is familiar with the three dimensions of color: hue, saturation, and brilliance. There is widespread confusion, though, about brilliance. *Brilliance* is the quality by which we distinguish a light col-

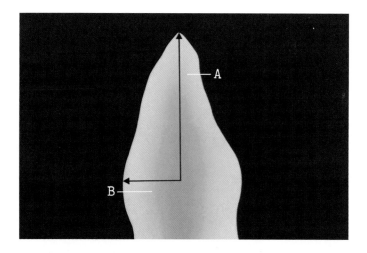

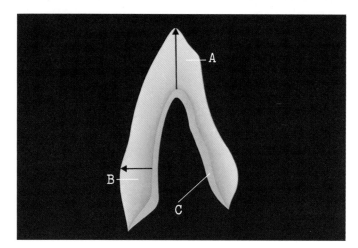

Figs 10-7 and 10-8 These schematic drawings illustrate the principle of a higher-saturated hue in the center blending to a lower-saturated one at the periphery. Figure 10-8 depicts the same principle for a metal ceramic crown. It is advisable to structure the layering of porcelain according to this method in order to find the correct color even under conditions of minimum thickness. *(A)* From the more saturated to the lighter hue; *(B)* from the more saturated to the lighter hue; *(C)* metal substructure.

or from a dark one. It is represented by the achromatic axis in the center of Munsell's cylinder, where white is at the top and black at the bottom (see Fig 1-6). There is a scale of grays ranging gradually from black to white and thus connecting the two extremes. Black has zero brilliance whereas white shows maximum brilliance.

If transparent and incisal porcelains are used, which are nuanced merely in gradations of gray, only gray teeth can be the result. For that reason, we prefer porcelain powders by Ivoclar. They contain more light

and less gray colors. Moreover, they provide a large range of translucencies that are distinguishable not only by their brilliance but by different hues as well (Fig 10-13):

− Slightly opalescent translucency (T1)
− Slightly pink translucency (T2)
− Slightly grayer translucency (T3)
− Highly transparent (T4)

These nuances can also be found on the palette of incisal porcelains. Consequently, it is simple for the ceramist to use these colors and subtleties without making the teeth unnecessarily gray (Fig 10-14).

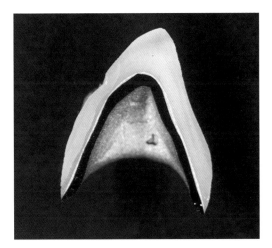

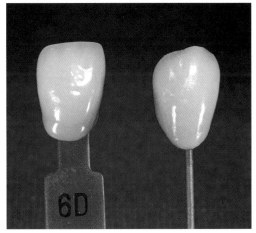

Fig 10-9 Again, a higher saturated hue can be seen in the center and a lower saturated one at the periphery of a metal ceramic crown. The clearly discernible transparent material has been applied beneath the incisal porcelain. The dentin color saturation decreases toward the surface (thickness of the dentin layer is 1 mm). The overall thickness of the restoration is 1.5 mm (metal coping, opaque, porcelain).

Fig 10-10 The same restoration as in Fig 10-9, prior to sectioning. The selected color 6D could be used although the thickness of the restoration did not exceed 1 mm. The opaque core is not visible. The main objective of this method is to create a maximum sense of depth in a restoration of minimum thickness.

Figs 10-11 and 10-12 Build-up and lateral segmentation techniques are complementary and result in very satisfying restorations. The object of study is an all-ceramic restoration. *(A)* Vanilla-colored "halo-effect," B-HY7; *(B)* transparent zone T4; *(C)* root portion B-HY3 + B-LB5; *(D)* transparent brown B-DB7; *(E)* vanilla-colored enamel cracks 101 + 104; *(F)* opalescent zones ID2 + DO3; *(G)* gray-brown beneath a layer of enamel porcelain B-DB3.

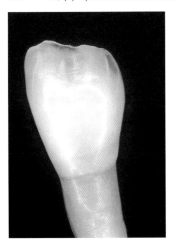

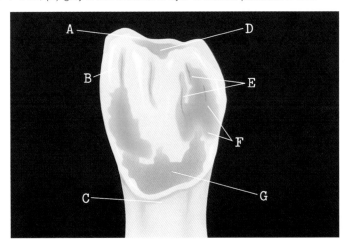

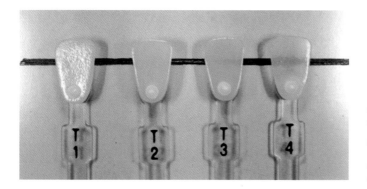

Fig 10-13 Transparent and translucent porcelains of the Ivoclar IPS Classic assortment. This assortment consists not only of colors of different brilliance but of different hues, too. Slightly opalescent transparent-porcelain (T1), a more pink porcelain (T2), a more gray porcelain (T3), and a very transparent porcelain (T4).

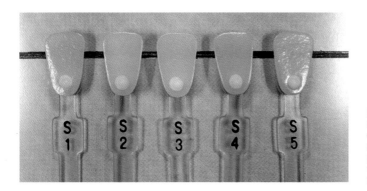

Fig 10-14 For transparent material and for the incisal porcelain also, colors of different brilliance are available. Thus it is possible to experiment with these color nuances without fabricating teeth that are unnecessarily gray.

Another unique aspect of the ceramics by Ivoclar is the "maverick" set. This set consists of four specially selected basic colors frequently found in natural teeth (Figs 10-15 to 10-18). Each of the four is created stepwise in three, five, and seven portions, desaturated with a neutral powder, thus forming four color groups (Figs 10-19 to 10-22). These mixtures are ready for use and are nuanced like natural material. They can readily be used during the build-up of ceramic layers, beginning with higher saturated colors and finishing with less saturated colors; they may further be used to provide a restoration with a characteristic touch (Figs 10-11, 10-12, 10-23, and 10-24).

In order to illustrate clearly the layering technique and laboratory procedures of these powders, a metal ceramic crown for a molar was fabricated. For better comprehen-

sion each step will be presented separately. Of course, full crown contour in porcelain is usually done as a one-step procedure with just one firing.

The main goal of the incremental build-up technique is to *create a sense of maximum depth and concurrently minimum thickness.* The application of only one dentin porcelain of a uniform degree of saturation "retards" the light suddenly, whereas light is "retarded" gradually if the layering technique is used; it enhances this sense of depth without disclosing the opaque porcelain core.

Firing of covering gold (Fig 10-25). This material is always applied when metal ceramic restorations are fabricated in order to avoid any gray reflection from underneath the opaque (see Fig 10-26).

Application of the first layer of highly saturated dentin porcelain and orange dentin

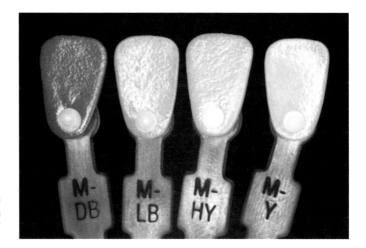

Fig 10-15 The four basic colors of the "maverick" porcelain set. These colors are less saturated and offer various possibilities.

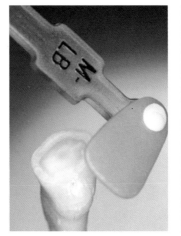

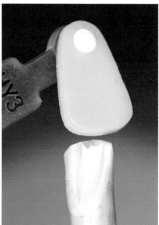

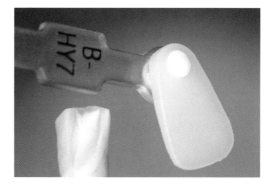

Figs 10-16 to 10-18 These pure and desaturated original colors often correspond with nuances of natural teeth.

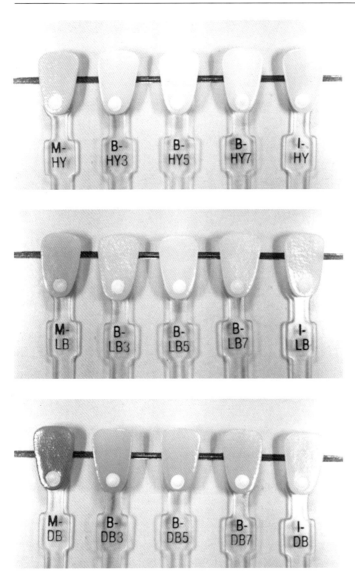

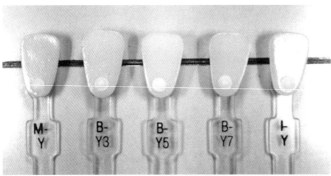

Figs 10-19 to 10-22 Each of the four basic colors of the maverick set is desaturated with a neutral powder in a gradation of three, five, and seven portions. The hue is always identical; not so the saturation. With regard to color selection, it is easier for the ceramist to use these pre-made reference colors than to mix them by himself or herself. The shade facets I-Y, I-LB, and I-HY are translucent colors derived from the basic colors. They are well suitable as incisal colors (see chapter 13, "Transparency and Translucency").

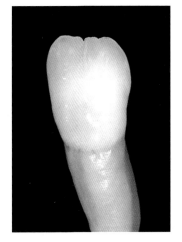
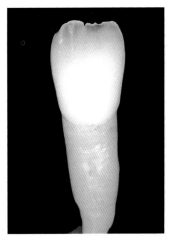

Fig 10-23 and 10-24 All-ceramic teeth. The maverick powders exhibit a minimal amount of saturation and are the material of choice for characterizing incisal edges and creating micro effects.

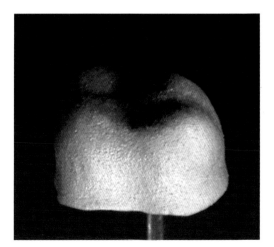

Fig 10-25 The fabrication of metal ceramic crowns inevitably involves the application of a covering gold layer.

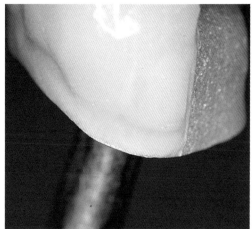

Fig 10-26 Because the covering gold was applied to the substructure, the cervical margin has a yellow-gold color. These areas would appear merely gray without the covering gold coat.

porcelain onto the proximal and occlusal surfaces (Fig 10-26). This simulates the color of the pulp, which acts iridescent in this region. This first layer of dentin porcelain is applied onto the opaque and, because it is the most saturated hue, should encompass the coping entirely. It is thought to mask the substructure, rendering it less "penetrable" than the other layers of dentin porcelain. The applied powder is one of the opaque dentin por-

celains by Ivoclar. However, the term opaque does not seem to be appropriate; we prefer the term "masking." These masking dental porcelains are well balanced with regard to the effects they create (ie, covering the opaque without changing the appearance of the restoration to opaque). Furthermore, they correspond with virtually every color of the Ivoclar set (for instance: opaque dentin mass 1D, 1C, 1E, etc).

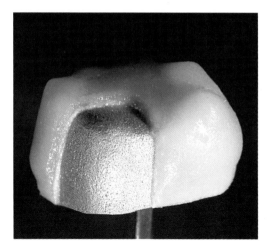

Fig 10-27   The firings have been performed in successive order for this study object. Normally the following steps are carried out at the same time, of course; usually one firing prior to the glaze bake will suffice. The first layer of a saturated dentin porcelain has been applied as has an orange dentin material onto the proximal and occlusal surfaces.

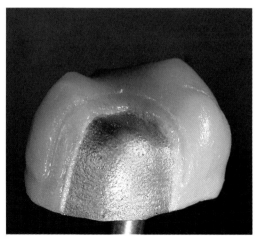

Fig 10-28   The second and slightly less saturated dentin porcelain has been applied.

This type of porcelain is particularly useful in the case of inadequate reduction. In a situation of minimum space, these porcelains allow masking of the substructure's opaque core without altering the basic color selected. In difficult situations with very little space, the first layer is also the thickest. If in the past we had to mask the substructure, and under-reduction was the problem, opaque dentin porcelains of a different color than the selected basic color were used. The substructure was masked in this way, but two significant risks had to be taken. First, these porcelains were too opaque and gave the restoration a "dull" appearance. Second, the overall color of the final restoration was not the selected basic color but exhibited exactly the color of the opaque dentin porcelains.

Application of the second, slightly less saturated dentin porcelain (Fig 10-28). Note there is neither cracking nor detachment in the periphery, even though no condensation was brought about. The cause for that is a grain-size reduction of 23% for the IPS powder. Mechanical condensation would have altered the desired surface roughness to a smooth finish. This second layer of dentin porcelain now exhibits the selected dentin color (eg, dentin 1D). It is the thickest of all three layers of dentin porcelain covering the entire restoration.

Application of the third layer, a mix of basic color dentin porcelain and 50% of the neutral dentin mass I-D1 (Fig 10-29). This layer is of lowest saturation, allowing the highest degree of light "penetration," because it is almost translucent. The mix must fully cover the restoration yet thin out toward the periphery. Low-saturated dentin porcelain causes a color to appear lighter. It is therefore significant to maintain the thickness of the first, more saturated layer. This third layer then compensates for color discrepancies and adapts well to the initially selected basic color.

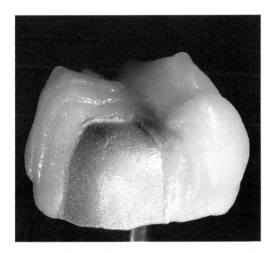

Fig 10-29 The third dentin layer, which exhibits the highest saturation, has been applied. This layer is a mix of basic color dentin porcelain and 50% of the neutral dentin mass ID1. Therefore this layer is most penetrable by light.

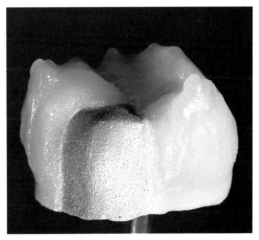

Fig 10-30 The transparent porcelain has been applied, incorporating some characterizations that are placed underneath the layer of incisal porcelain. These colors are applied with the lateral segmentation technique.

Example: hue 1D (Figs 10-33 and 10-34)

– First dentin layer: opaque dentin mass 1D; thickness ± 1/4 of all three layers
– Second dentin layer: dentin mass 1D; thickness ± 2/4 of all three layers
– Third dentin layer: dentin mass 1D, desaturated with 50% of a neutral mass; thickness ± 1/4 of all three layers

Application of transparent porcelain and characterization of colors according to lateral segmentation technique (Fig 10-30).

Application of incisal porcelain according to lateral segmentation technique (Fig 10-31). In order to complete my range of colors and to achieve a restoration more vital in appearance, custom-made incisal colors such as mother-of-pearl, opalescent, and vanilla are applied (see chapter 14 "Original Colors in Dental Ceramics").

Following is a description of the technique we apply to build up and imitate natural-looking teeth. If no low-saturated porcelain is commercially available, it should be custom mixed, always bearing in mind that the initial dentin layer should exhibit a more saturated hue than the selected basic color. The other dentin layers, which should exhibit less color saturation, consist of a mix of dentin porcelain and the neutral mass I-D1. That material does not change the color brilliance of a tooth at all. The technique is also applicable for the fabrication of all-ceramic inlays and onlays (Fig 10-32).

This technique, commencing with an opaque core, involves an incremental build-up from highly saturated to less saturated colors to create a restoration with a sense of maximum depth and minimal thickness. Furthermore, the incisal porcelain is superimposed on the transparent porcelain, and masking dentin porcelain is used instead of porcelains that are opaque and may deleteriously affect the restoration's natural appearance.

Once again, we would like to emphasize

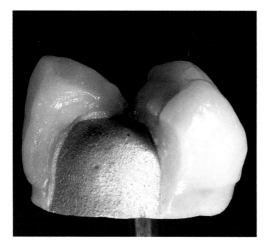

Fig 10-31 Modeling of the restoration is completed with the application of an opalescent incisal porcelain.

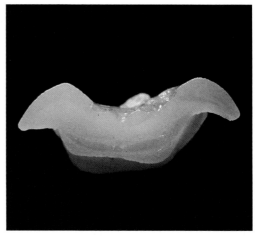

Fig 10-32 The layering technique, progressing from the most saturated to the lightest color, can also be used for ceramic inlays and onlays. This cross section of an inlay clearly depicts the applied method.

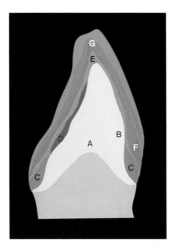

Fig 10-33 Build-up of a metal ceramic crown following the principle of layering from the highest saturation to the lightest colors. (A) Substructure; (B) opaque; (C) opaque dentin; (D) orange to mimic the color of the pulp; this orange color is applied to the proximal surface to act as an iridescent and create an orange reflection, thus imitating the pulp of a natural tooth; (E) dentin porcelain, which masks the most saturated porcelain; (F) basic material of the selected color; (G) dentin porcelain that is desaturated with 50% of a neutral mass.

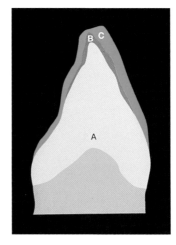

Fig 10-34 Layering of the transparent and incisal porcelains. (A) Dentin core; (B) transparent porcelain that has been applied beneath the incisal layer for reasons of light circulation; (C) incisal porcelain that is an equivalent to the enamel of a natural tooth.

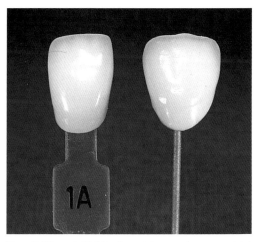
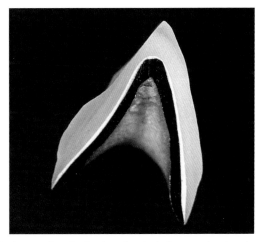

Figs 10-35 and 10-36 A metal ceramic crown fabricated according to the layering technique and using the shade 1A. Although the thickness of the restoration (metal, opaque, and porcelain) is only 1.5 mm, its color matches the selected one well without allowing the opaque core to shine through.

that our conclusions are based on observations of nature, tooth sections, and natural teeth. This technique may serve as an aid in difficult cases. At first it may seem as if this approach implies a certain amount of coercion; however, this feeling disappears once the technique has been assimilated in laboratory practice and will consequently result in close similarity to nature (Figs 10-35 to 10-42).

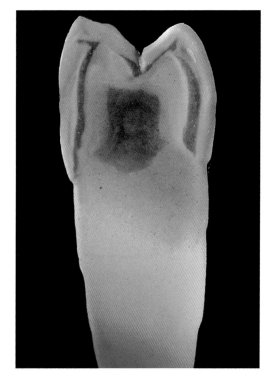

Fig 10-37 All-ceramic tooth for study. Every ceramist who is prepared to learn and improve his or her skill should work with cross sections. The authors regard this method as compulsory for better comprehension.

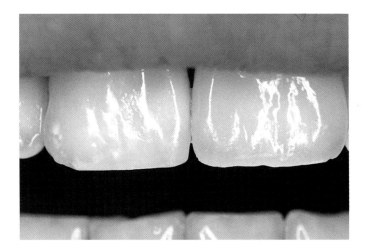

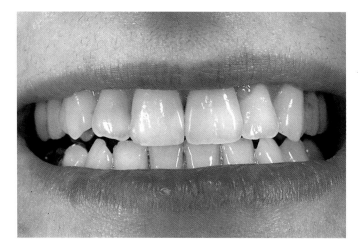

Figs 10-38 and 10-39 Metal ceramic crown on tooth 21. (Courtesy of Dr Michel Roge, Béziers, France.)

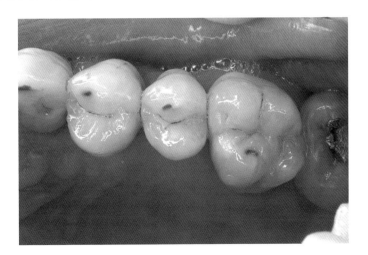

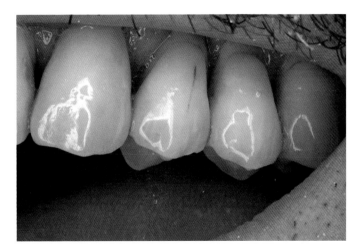

Figs 10-40 and 10-41 Metal ceramic fixed partial denture from tooth 13 to tooth 16 (replacement of tooth 15). Note the rotation of the pontic of tooth 15, which gives the fixed partial denture a natural appearance. (Courtesy of Dr Daniel Gleyzolle, Avignon, France.)

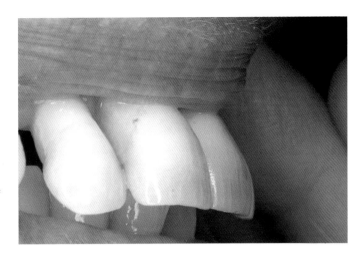

Fig 10-42 Metal ceramic crown on tooth 11. Note the incorporation of enamel cracks, which adapts well to the adjacent natural tooth 21. (Courtesy of Dr Thierry Jeannin, Orange, France.)

Table of Firing Temperatures

It is difficult to specify exact temperatures for firing procedures because different porcelains require different manipulations. A wide variety of furnaces and commercial products are available. Prior to a discussion about firing temperatures, some parameters of considerable significance for our objective must be specified. The following describes the important points of reference:

- Porcelain: IPS classic and "maverick" (Ivoclar)
- Furnace: Ivoclar P.90 (well calibrated)
- No condensation of porcelain during procedures
- Creamy consistency of porcelain during modeling

Programs	Start temperature	Heating (rate/min)	Drying	Vacuum start	Vacuum end	Holding time	Final temperature
Opaque-wash	400°	80°	2 min	600°	950°	–	950°
Covering gold (Keradec Wieland)	400°	60°	5 min	600°	820°	–	820°
Opaque	400°	80°	4 min	600°	950°	–	950°
Shoulder porcelain 1st and 2nd firing	400°	60°	5 min	600°	949°	1 min	950°
1st bisque bake	400°	60°	9 min	600°	919°	1 min	920°
2nd bisque bake	400°	60°	5 min	600°	899°	1 min	900°
Minimum glaze bake	400°	60°	2 min	–	–	1 min	890°
Glaze and correction bake	400°	60°	5 min	600°	889°	1 min	890°

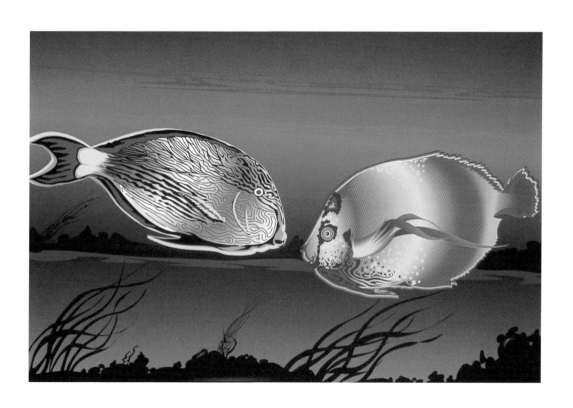

11 Tricks to Make Porcelain Layering Easier

Fabrication of a Multi-Span Fixed Partial Denture

In order to achieve a satisfactory esthetic result, we prefer to split the fabrication procedure in several sections, ie, we focus on the anterior region first. The procedure is staged as follows:

① **First bake:** fabrication of the anterior segment (six teeth) (Fig 11-1)

② **Second bake:** fabrication of the posterior segments and correction of the anterior segment (Fig 11-2)

③ **Third bake:** correction of the posterior segments and correction of the anterior segment if necessary (Fig 11-3)

Glaze bake: vacuum firing for minor corrections; polishing for completion

If the restoration is to be a long-span fixed partial denture, the application of the porcelain in one step should be done for study purposes only. In general, one-step layering is detrimental for the porcelain and may lower the overall quality of the restoration. It reduces our ability to create effects that can only be created with internal staining. Therefore, we prefer to section the fabrication procedure (Fig 11-4).

Fabrication in stages has two advantages: *the procedure is easier and it enables the technician to create a highly esthetic restoration according to the following three significant parameters:*

1. Rapid modeling
2. Ability to maintain a constant degree of moisture
3. No condensation of porcelain

Fabrication of Anterior Fixed Partial Dentures

Our attention must be focused entirely on the restoration at hand and the three parameters mentioned above must be permanently considered. The ceramic layering begins with the labial surfaces in order to perfectly mimic the complex effects. After completion of the labial surfaces we proceed to the lingual areas. This is all performed before the first firing (Figs 11-5 and 11-6).

It may prove necessary in certain difficult cases to bake the labial build-up first and successively fire the lingual surface and then perform final labial corrections.

Layering and Firing of the "Dentin" Core

A different approach is used in cases of unusually delicately characterized anterior teeth: first the dentin porcelain is applied and all effects, even the transparent ones, are created, then the unfinished restoration is fired. Immediately afterwards we can assess both color and function. This method of layering allows for accurate control of the internal (dentin) porcelain layers and correction if

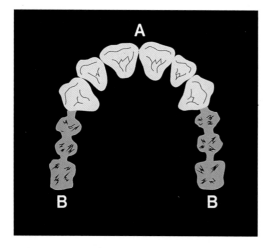

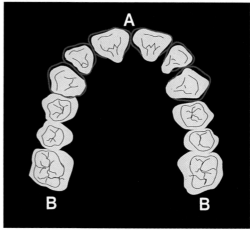

Figs 11-1 to 11-13 Fabrication of a multi-span fixed partial denture.

Fig 11-1 First the anterior segment *(A)* is modeled and fired: *first bake.*

Fig 11-2 The posterior segments *(B)* are fabricated in a second step while the anterior segment *(A)* is simultaneously corrected: *second bake.*

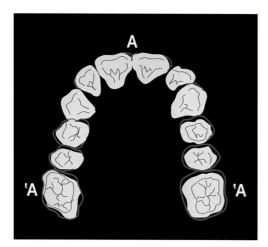

Fig 11-3 The third step involves correction of the posterior segments *('A)* while the contour of the anterior segment *(A)* is touched-up if needed: *third bake.*

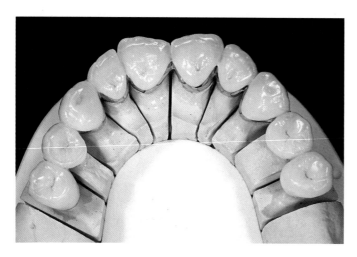

Fig 11-4 Example of a metal ceramic fixed partial denture that has been fabricated according to the above-mentioned procedures.

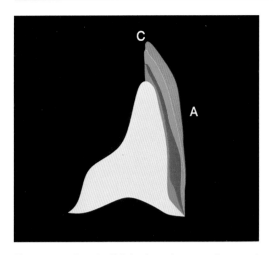
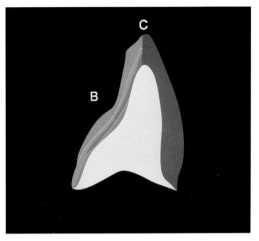

Figs 11-5 and 11-6 Fabrication of crowns for anterior teeth in two steps: *(1)* build-up of all labial surfaces in accordance to the layering technique and the principle of lateral segmentation; *(2)* build-up of the lingual surfaces. Obviously, esthetics are of major significance concerning anterior teeth. Therefore, we must concentrate particularly on the labial surfaces during the procedure. The entire esthetic result depends on the layering and the segmentation of the labial surfaces. The ceramist should not concentrate on the lingual surface and functional aspects until this important step is completed.

Figs 11-7 to 11-10 If anterior teeth are to be restored and delicate effects within the tooth are important, the first part to be built up is the dentin core and all desired effects; even transparent porcelain is applied at this stage. A first firing follows and in the second step the incisal porcelain can be applied.

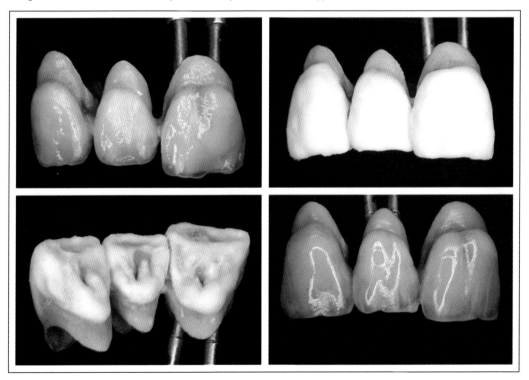

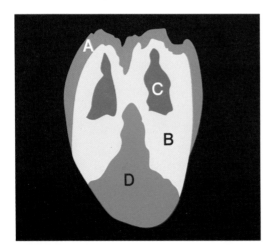

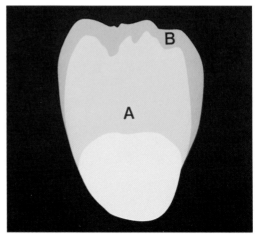

Fig 11-11 Fabrication of a metal ceramic restoration. First the dentin core and the transparent zone are built up and fired. This method facilitates the perfect positioning of porcelain layers within the restoration and proper control after the firing. *(A)* Transparent porcelain; *(B)* dentin porcelain; *(C)* mamelon effects; *(D)* dentin porcelains of different saturation and hue.

Fig 11-12 After the bake of the dentire core with all effects and the transparent zone, the position and function are inspected, as is the space that must ultimately be provided for the incisal build-up. *(A)* Layering of the incisal porcelain; *(B)* transparent porcelain applied beneath the incisal porcelain.

necessary. Only when the second firing is performed is the incisal porcelain applied, thus completing the build-up (Figs 11-7 to 11-10). This method is also used for the lighter hues and positioning of transparent zones (Figs 11-11 and 11-12).

Density of Porcelain During Layering Procedure

In order to facilitate the layering and to secure the porcelain slurry in its position during modeling, the initial material must be dense and compact. The successive layers, however, should be less dense and softer, otherwise the layer beneath could be subjected to undesirable shifting. Application will be facilitated considerably if the incisal porcelain is of an almost liquid consistency. In brief, the basic mass should be dense and compact,

then becoming softer to almost liquid at completion. For this purpose, a premium-quality liquid is used to maintain a creamy consistency of the ceramic and thus preventing a breakdown of the build-up (Fig 11-13).

Another Trick: Grinding the Incisal Guidance

In order to correctly adjust and grind the incisal guiding path of two antagonistic fixed partial dentures, a 50-μm aluminum paste (Fig 11-14) is applied to the questionable incisal edges. All mandibular motions are simulated in the articulator. The paste is abrasive and grinds the guiding area of the articulating motion (Fig 11-15). The points of contact must be totally congruent. The roughened surface of the porcelain must be repolished after the grinding process (Fig 11-16).

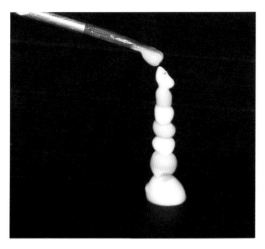

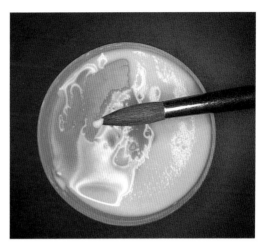

Fig 11-13 A premium-quality liquid is used for the modeling procedure. It maintains a creamy consistency and prevents breakdown of the build-up (liquid N, Ivoclar).

Fig 11-14 Water/aluminum paste mix, grain size 50 μm.

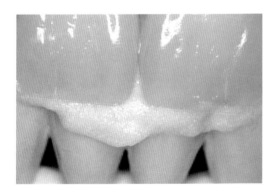

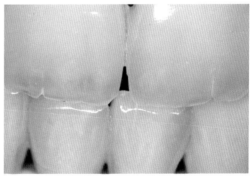

Figs 11-15 and 11-16 The aluminum paste acts as an abrasive. It facilitates the optimum adjustment of functional incisal sliding areas. Note that the porcelain must be repolished with diamond polishing paste to smooth the roughened surface.

12   Lateral Segmentation and Enamel Cracks

In retrospect, my early ceramic restorations were remarkably simpler regarding the build-up of porcelain layers. In those days, application of the new material did not allow time to experiment with special effects. I doubted whether it would ever be feasible to imitate nature and create the illusion of a natural tooth with ceramic restorations. Willi Geller was the first dental technician whose work imitated naturalness close to "perfection."

Willi Geller doubtlessly represented one of the first who used his outstanding abilities of observation and application to create restorations that closely matched the original. His lateral segmentation technique seems as if directly derived from the layering technique. Today it appears difficult to fabricate natural restorations that seem to be "alive." The most

complex part of a metal ceramic restoration certainly is the incisal third of an anterior tooth. Details are more subtle and colors more discrete and translucent in this region, thus creating additional problems. The vital appearance of anterior crowns depends to a great deal on the design of the incisal edge. It seems to be the zone of the imperceptible characterization. But here, too, the interplay of shape and color contributes to a natural appearance (Fig 12-1).

Lateral segmentation is a vertical build-up of ceramic segments varying in brilliance, translucency, and color. This method is used for older as well as younger patients.

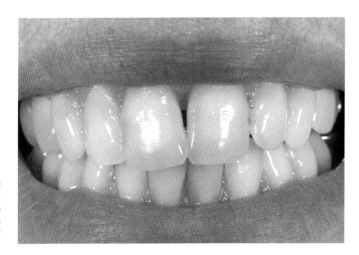

Fig 12-1 The most esthetic part of human teeth is the maxillary incisal edge. It represents the most intricate area to be reproduced – the details are more subtle and the shades are more discrete and translucent.

Restoration and Segmentation for Teeth of Older Patients

In the teeth of older patients, color and brilliance contrast quite distinctly, and enamel cracks act as discernible demarcation for each segment. When we prepare the different mixtures for our palette with the intention of using different incisal colors, the variety of brilliance and hue becomes predictable: slighly blueish, more opalescent, grayish, or more reddish (S1, S2, S3, S4 of the Ivoclar set). When a fixed partial denture for the anterior region is to be fabricated, I prefer to apply a slighly blueish incisal color to the proximal area. The grayest segments are located in the center. The segments with more opalescent, lighter incisal colors are located discretely in between. In order to imitate one single tooth, we reproduce only the different nuances and their location within the tooth.

The transparent porcelain applied to the incisal edge (see chapter 10, "Processing and Natural Build-up of Dental Porcelain") is a combination of various hues. We are not reluctant to use a whole set of different transparent porcelains (T1, T2, T3, T4 by Ivoclar); these respective porcelains are slightly pink, blueish, more gray, and somewhat opalescent, and they enable us to create a slight lateral segmentation during application. The Maverick transparent porcelain set serves as an aid, too. These subtle color additions do not need to be conspicuous, but they supply the ceramic restoration with a vital appearance.

Segments of Different Opacity

During application of the incisal porcelain the translucency of the segments is usually varied. It is possible to mix dentin porcelain with 50% of a neutral porcelain (eg, ID1, Ivoclar) or an opaque dentin porcelain with a neutral one (ratio always 1:1). These segments are more opaque and mask and

influence the light in a "retarding" manner. However, these streaks are usually smaller and represent overlaid oxides to create enamel cracks.

Restoration and Segmentation for Teeth of Younger Patients

Lateral segmentation of teeth for younger patients is identical to that for older patients, with the only change being amount. The nuances in color, brilliance, and translucency are more subtle and discrete. Once the restoration is completed, the segments will no longer be distinguishable. A large number of effects, however, create a vital appearance of the porcelain.

When using this lateral segmentation technique, the positioning of the segments must not be similar to that of piano keys. Their dimensions and widths are not determined by a general rule, nor is their shape totally parallel or right-angled. The restoration should be logical but without the rigidity of a machine or an instrument.

Segmentation of Posterior Teeth

Lateral segmentation is also used for posterior teeth. The basic shape of the tooth is established first (the occlusal surfaces or occlusion itself are not yet considered). We begin with the labial portion and work gradually around the tooth (Figs 12-2 and 12-3). When the modeling of the basic shape is completed, we fabricate the occlusal surfaces and occlusal contacts.

This technique is appropriate particularly for the fabrication of large fixed partial dentures. While we focus initially on the direction of the restorative process and then apply, step by step, the ceramic segments, a constant coefficient of moisture must be maintained. During the fabrication of fixed partial dentures, the problem of drying of the porcelain occurs. If we apply the ceramic

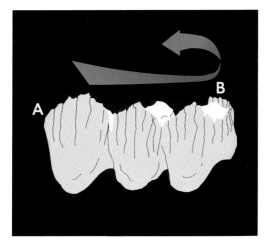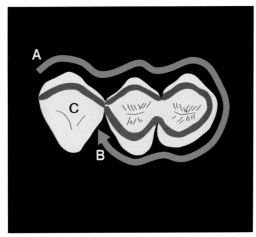

Figs 12-2 and 12-3 The layering of the incisal edges of fixed partial dentures and crowns is performed by means of the lateral segmentation technique. First, we begin at the mesial side of the labial portion and proceed gradually around the tooth to the point where we started from. Layering according to this method offers one major advantage: the ceramic material maintains a constant degree of moisture without any alteration. Moisture is thus gradually transported during layering of the segments. If we succeed in maintaining this constant degree of moisture during the entire process, a key step in achieving a pleasant esthetic result has been done.

in just one direction, it will be possible to maintain moisture while working our way around the restoration. A constant degree of moisture is crucial for vital-appearing restorations and high-quality porcelain.

Modeling Criteria for Porcelain of Superior Optic Quality

Three criteria must be met for a successful imitation of the vital appearance of a natural tooth.

First criterion: the porcelain must be homogeneous and not too liquid; the ceramic slurry must retain a certain shape when lifted by the point of the brush (Fig 12-4).

Second criterion: the porcelain must be applied as rapidly as possible to avoid drying. Nothing adversely affects porcelain more than drying and repeated wetting; layering carried out in that manner results in a restoration devoid of any vital appearance.

Third criterion: forceful condensation should be avoided; it would result in a color shift and an undesirable mix-up of all effects previously created with great care. Furthermore, the condensed porcelain would be of lower quality after firing, because the material would appear less penetrable by light. According to the "rule of colors" in painting, shifting and mixing render the restoration grayer.

The above criteria are the keys to success. If they are ignored, the inevitable result will be a lifeless restoration.

Enamel Cracks

Thorough observation of natural teeth discloses, particularly during shade selection procedures, the common characteristic of enamel cracks (Fig 12-5). These cracks are generally delicate and light-colored in young teeth, more numerous and darker-colored in older teeth.

It is necessary to mimic these minute

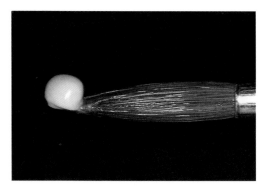

Fig 12-4 The porcelain must be homogeneous and have a creamy consistency. A constant degree of moisture must be maintained throughout the application procedure.

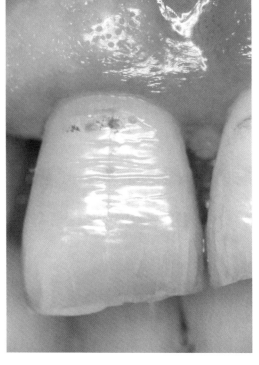

Fig 12-5 If this tooth were to be restored, it would be necessary to incorporate numerous enamel cracks. The largest cracks are at the transitions to the proximal surfaces. Note the differently angulated directions of the cracks.

defects, otherwise the ceramic restoration could be taken for the replica of a natural tooth merely by name and not because of appearance. Cracks convey the illusion of increased depth. The technique of lateral segmentation makes the fabrication relatively simple.

Figure 12-6 shows a central incisor with numerous cracks and light discolorations. Every effect and color characteristic has been imitated. For the purpose of copying tooth 11, it was unnecessary to stain the surface. When the shade was selected, every feature of the cracks was recorded in a scheme (Fig 12-7). The incisal third shows darker and wider cracks than the proximal portion. In the center, on the other hand, the cracks are white, creamy, and more delicate.

In the subdivision of the porcelain being used for our restoration, it is obvious that the

schematic distribution of the ceramic is identical with the case. This may be different with another clinical case (Figs 12-8 and 12-9).

A well-defined streak of brown is applied to the incisal third. It consists of equal portions of dentin porcelain 2A, an intense brown ID6 and orange ID3. This is covered by a precisely defined layer of gray underlaid with a translucent gray T3. Two of the dentin porcelains are important: a particularly light dentin porcelain 2A in the center as well as a less light but rather yellow dentin 1C in the cervical third. The distinctly defined marginal area is built up using shoulder porcelain M3 and M4 (ratio 3/4 : 1/4).

Inside the oral cavity these cracks function like a vehicle for light and the phenomenon of refraction renders them visible; light seems to "paint" the walls of these microfissures. Figure 12-10 shows the influence of light on these cracks: viewed from different angles

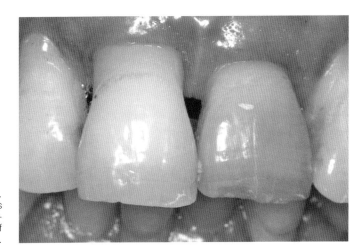

Fig 12-6 Tooth 21 is to be restored. The adjacent tooth shows numerous enamel cracks. For reasons of perfect adaptation, the technique of lateral segmentation should be used.

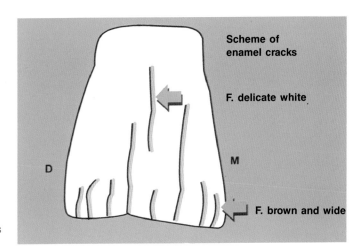

Scheme of enamel cracks

F. delicate white

D

M

F. brown and wide

Fig 12-7 Scheme of characteristics of enamel cracks.

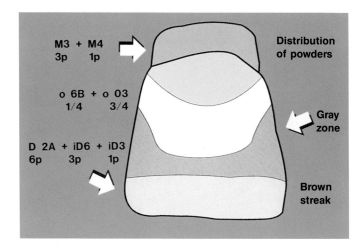

Fig 12-8 Different porcelain powders are chosen during the shade selection process.

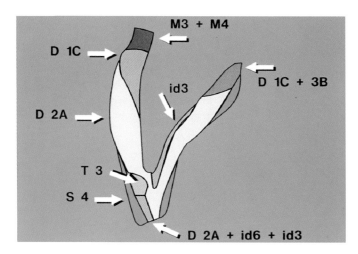

Fig 12-9 Positioning of the ceramic powders especially selected for the individual clinical case shown. The distribution must be adapted to each individual case.

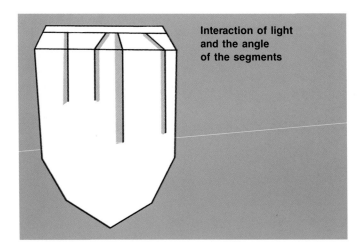

Fig 12-10 Light moves according to the angle of the segments, altering their appearance from wide to less wide.

Fig 12-11 *(left)* The crack appears fine when viewed directly. It is a 90º angle to the surface of the glass.

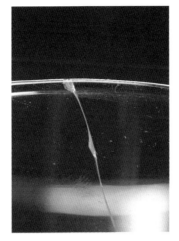
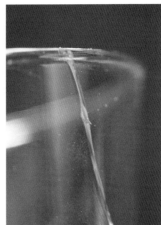

Fig 12-12 *(right)* The crack appears wider when viewed from an angle more oblique to the crack.

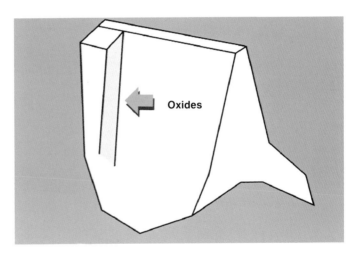

Oxides

Fig 12-13 Effect colors (metal oxides) are applied to the stress-bearing segment.

the cracks apparently vary in width. A photograph of a cracked glass may serve as an aid for better understanding this effect that light has on enamel cracks (Figs 12-11 and 12-12). This is the principle we must adhere to for the creation of cracks in porcelain. Instead of light "painting" the walls of a crack, it is the ceramist who applies metal oxides to the walls of the stress-bearing segments (Fig 12-13).

Cracks created in porcelain are artificial and we have to use staining colors to attain these effects (Fig 12-14). Metal oxides are prepared in a saturated mix (Fig 12-15). The

oxides are applied with the small, flat marten's hair brush no. 2. Prior to each application it is absolutely necessary to rinse and clean the brush (a fingernail may be used as a mini palette). It is advisable to create an almost invisible crack, otherwise the crown may appear unrealistic. The metal oxides are applied to the stress-bearing segment, working from the incisal edge to the cervical region (Fig 12-16). There should be no second application, because this would create too big a crack. To make a crack clearly visible, the angle of the stress-bearing segment is

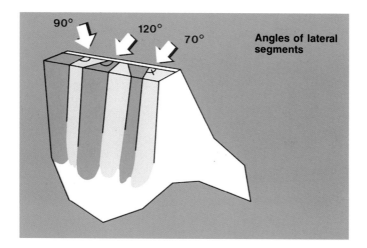

Fig 12-14 A variety of widths can serve as an aid to give the lateral segments different angles.

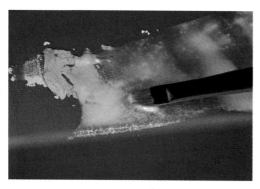

Fig 12-15 The effect colors are toned down while they are mixed. The saturation must be adapted to the crack.

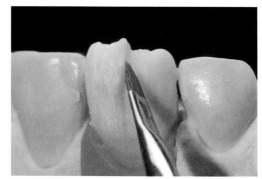

Fig 12-16 A small, flat brush is used for the staining. The crack is "painted" in an incisocervical direction.

increased (120°) (Fig 12-17), and a transparent segment is superimposed on the structure to act as a filter, similar to a fiberoptic lens and thus making the crack conspicuous. This type of wider crack is usually found in the proximal portion of teeth.

When fine and discrete cracks are created, the angle of the stress-bearing segment should be 90° (Fig 12-18). The porcelain applied to that structure should be a masking layer and act like a filter. A mix of dentin porcelain or an opaque "dentin" and a neutral porcelain is generally used. The penetrating light is "retard-

ed" and the semiopacity of the segment conceals the wall that is covered by metal oxides. Consequently, the crack appears more delicate. Working with a variety of segment angles requires little experience and can be quite satisfying in the attempt to copy nature.

The clinical result of the presented case is one such satisfying example (Figs 12-19 and 12-20). All in all, it shows that if enamel cracks are a characteristic of natural teeth, they should be included in the restorations (Figs 12-21 to 12-23).

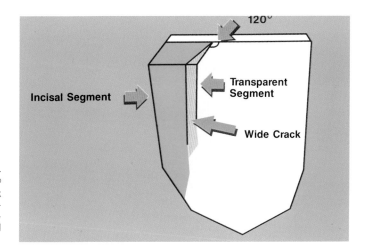

Fig 12-17 The stress-bearing segment here shows an angle of 135° (ie, wide open); thus, the crack appears wide. To make this characteristic salient, a segment of transparent material must be superimposed on the underlying staining colors.

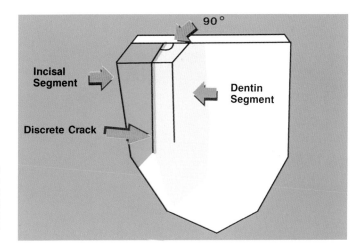

Fig 12-18 If the crack is to be delicate and discrete, the stress-bearing segment must exhibit an angle of 90°. The segment that superimposes upon the staining colors must be masking and must "retard" the light.

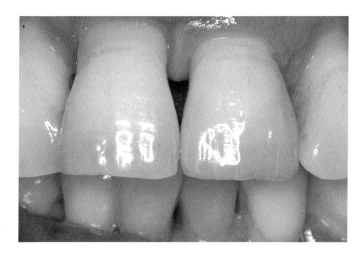

Fig 12-19 Tooth 21 has been restored with a metal ceramic crown. The crown, which has been fabricated according to the lateral segmentation technique and with incorporated enamel cracks, adapts perfectly to adjacent tooth 11. (Courtesy of Dr Thierry Jeannin, Orange, France.)

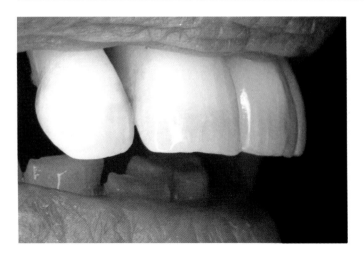

Fig 12-20 This view makes apparent the perfect mimicry of the enamel cracks incorporated in the metal ceramic crown.

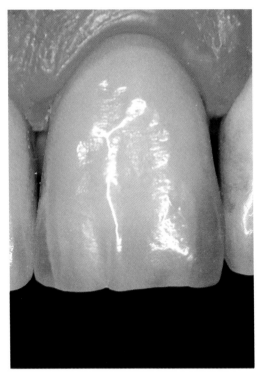

Fig 12-21 Another study of the incorporation of enamel cracks.

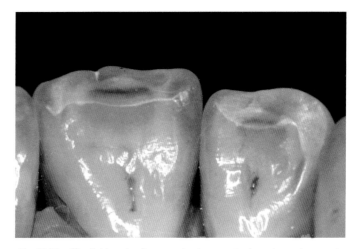

Fig 12-22   The flat brush allows ready characterization of a surface on the stress-bearing segment. The lingual view reveals the depths of the cracks, which are discernible on the abraded incisal edges.

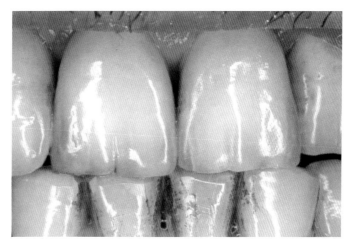

Fig 12-23   Teeth 11, 12, 13, 21, and 23 have been restored with metal ceramic crowns. (Clinical work by Dr Daniel Gleyzolle, Avignon, France.)

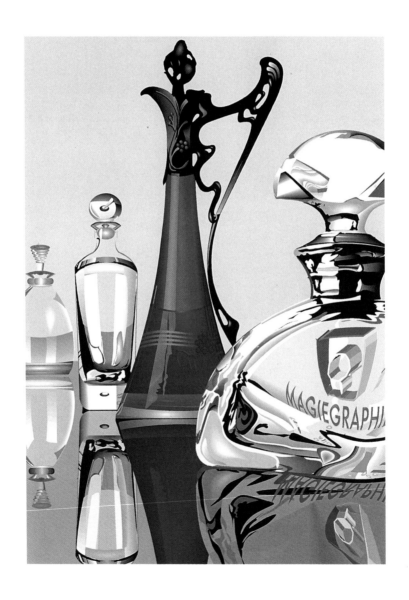

13 Transparency and Translucency

Transparency and translucency must not be confused. The use of these terms in communication between dentists and technicians requires that we be specific. The term transparency applies to material that allows light to penetrate, while objects behind still appear quite clear. No light is reflected on the surface of a transparent material.

The term translucency characterizes a material that does not allow the object behind to be readily visible. Light must thus be reflected to a certain extent and the material is of more opaque appearance.

Enamel. A tooth is entirely covered by enamel. The enamel is more or less translucent depending on the patient's age. Therefore, it is not logical to restore different teeth with the same translucent incisal porcelain. In addition, incisal edges incorporate numerous nuances of color and brilliance. Consequently, it would be incorrect to use just one incisal color for all teeth (Figs 13-1 to 13-5).

Transparency of a natural tooth. Natural teeth are rarely transparent; only very young teeth show transparent zones at their thin and long incisal edges, usually between the mamelons, at the far end of the incisal edge, and at the mesial and distal proximal surfaces. This transparency changes from gray to dark blue (Fig 13-6).

However, there are transparent zones in older patients' teeth, too. In general, these teeth show considerable wear because of a distinct overbite; this situation leads to very sharp-edged abrasion facets. This situation originates from the extreme overlap and the functional stress of the incisal edges. Dentin has almost completely vanished at the edges,

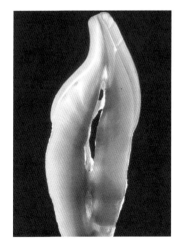 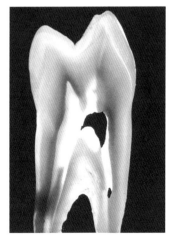

Figs 13-1 and 13-2 Cross sections of natural teeth. Note the considerable thickness of the enamel and the minor translucency.

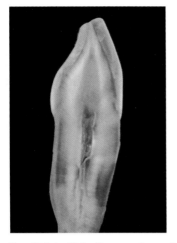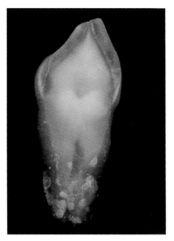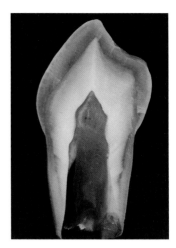

Figs 13-3 to 13-5 Cross sections of natural teeth. These teeth exhibit enamel of much higher translucency. The dentin shows translucent zones, too. These zones are not regular; they appear mainly in the periphery of the crown and in random display.

and the very thin enamel layer shows a glasslike appearance. The color ranges from gray to dark blue and is produced by the darkness of the oral cavity (Fig 13-7).

Working with transparent and translucent porcelains. Beginners in dental ceramics often misuse transparent porcelain, which can impart a glasslike appearance that exhibits too much gray. If, on top of that, a gray incisal color is used, most likely the entire restoration will be gray when completed. In order to avoid this "gray" mistake, colored transparent porcelain and multicolored incisal porcelain of varying translucency should be used.

Working with transparent material. This material must always be applied beneath the incisal porcelain, as explained in the discus-

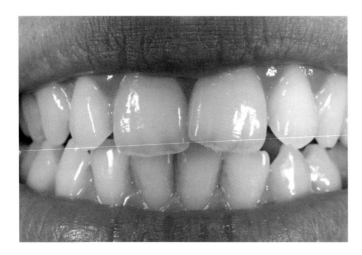

Fig 13-6 The incisal edges of anterior teeth in a young person show numerous subtle characteristics and appear very translucent.

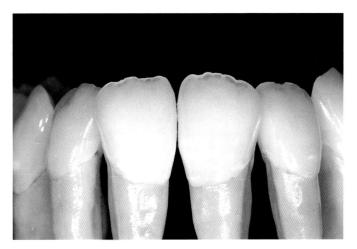

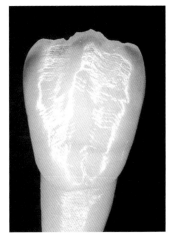

Fig 13-7 *(left)* An older tooth restored in ceramic with distinct, sharp wear facets because of a considerable overlap of the anterior teeth. The incisal edge, which is subjected to functional loading and therefore extremely thin, exhibits very transparent zones. The incisal porcelain is of a gray tinge and very translucent (2/3 neutral powder + 1/3 incisal powder).
(right) A rather bright tooth (all-ceramic restoration). The zones of transparency are quite conspicuous, too. The entire surface was built up using only one incisal porcelain.

Figs 13-8 and 13-9 All-ceramic restorations showing a distinct, dark blue, transparent seam (see chapter 14, "Original Colors in Dental Ceramics"). The incisal porcelain is semitranslucent (incisal powder S1 1/3 + 2/3 neutral powder).

sion of the layering technique. Yet the transparent zone varies in thickness. If the transparent layer is meant to be a distinct feature, greater amounts must be applied in a precisely specified manner. For example, the teeth of young patients with fine incisal edges are clearly transparent. In such cases, the transparent material must be applied in an exact manner. We prefer a material that reflects gray (T4 IPS/Ivoclar) or a dark blue transpa-

rent porcelain (see chapter 14, "Original Colors in Dental Ceramics"). If the material must imitate the appearance of a transparent incisal edge, it should not be applied over a large surface area onto the dentin porcelain. It would be advisable to cover the build-up with a layer of semitranslucent enamel porcelain (Figs 13-8 and 13-9).

In cases where transparency is desired to be inconspicuous (ie, only slightly visible

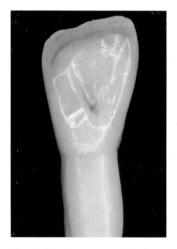
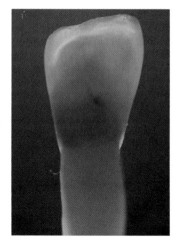
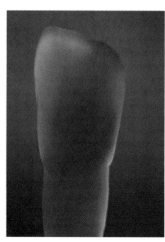

Fig 13-10 All-ceramic restorations. The transparent porcelain has been applied under the pure incisal porcelain.

Figs 13-11 and 13-12 The same tooth as in Fig 13-10, illuminated from behind. These figures clearly show that a pure incisal porcelain superimposed on the transparent porcelain can mask the transparent zone on the facial side. Light can now freely circulate inside the tooth.

underneath the enamel), I prefer to use a range of differently colored transparent porcelains and not just one of gray color if possible. These layers that cover the dentin porcelain thin out to the central region. The incisal porcelain instead should be less translucent and applied unaltered (S1, S2, S3, S4, S5) (Figs 13-10 to 13-12).

Use of translucent material for incisal edges. As we have discussed before, relating to the layering technique, it is not desirable to choose a single gray for the incisal build-up; rather a colored material should be chosen. Admittedly, however, a tooth's translucency is not always identical. Therefore, translucent colors should be used that match the color of a tooth to be restored. Our preferred set (S1, S2, S3, S4, S5) is reduced in saturation and altered to a higher translucency by mixing with the neutral powder ID1. The mixing ratio

generally is 2/3 incisal to 1/3 neutral powder or 1/2 to 1/2 or 1/3 to 2/3 incisal to neutral to obtain even more translucency. The translucent colors of the Maverick set are particularly good to work with. These basic colors, which are mixed with a neutral powder at a ratio of 1:7, are well dosed and serve as an aid to creating incisal color with yellow, honey-colored, light-colored, and dark-colored reflections (Fig 13-13). This set of translucent colors, which will be custom-made if needed, will always have to be a mix of a neutral powder with an "intense" or dentin powder.

These translucent colors fully cover the tooth, thus increasing the sense of depth (Figs 13-14 and 13-15). However, this technique requires remarkable experience in the field of dental ceramics. The student should use only "homeopathic" amounts in the beginning to avoid early discouragement.

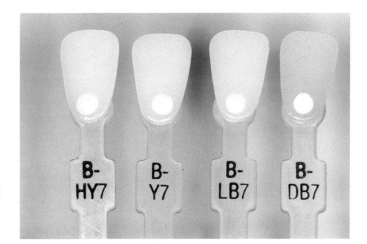

Fig 13-13 Translucent colors of the Maverick kit: honey, yellow, light brown, and dark brown. These translucent colors can be used for incisal edges as well as for subtle characterizations.

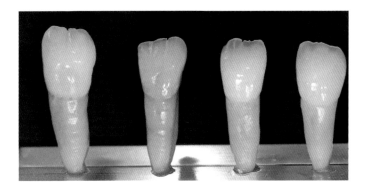

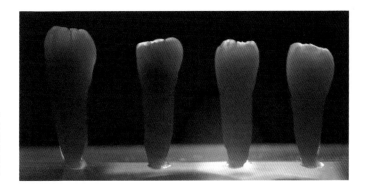

Figs 13-14 and 13-15 Further studies of all-ceramic objects which illustrate the possibilities transparent and translucent zones can offer. The extent of these zones depends on the shape and size of the tooth and the patient's age.

14 Original Colors in Dental Ceramics

At times even the most comprehensive-appearing set of dental porcelain colors may require a custom mix. The painter's palette is infinite, and the one a ceramist uses is enormous, too. For this reason, I have standardized certain colors. These colors are considered indispensable.

① **Slightly milky, opalescent porcelain.** This porcelain is used quite frequently today. Many teeth exhibit opalescent zones, particularly lighter colors. This well dosed color (Fig 14-1) is suitable to be used as dentin porcelain for the dentin core and as incisal porcelain for milky-white incisal edges. This opalescent material must contain a sufficient amount of white without creating too opaque an impression (Fig 14-2). This material is also used to form the summit of the cusp ridges and the mamelons. The mixing ratio of this material is as follows:
- 6 portions of the neutral powder ID1
- 1 portion of the white powder ID2.

② **Transparent, dark blue porcelain.** My set of translucent powders does not supply a dark blue. This particular color proves very useful when incisal edges of high transparency are built up (teeth of younger patients generally show this feature). The color is applied sparingly in quite distinct streaks confined to the incisal region (Fig 14-3). For delicate situations, where subtlety and precision are required, this effect may be secured by an advanced firing procedure, while the restoration will later be completed with an additional firing. The amount of this porcelain should not be too great in order to avoid any undesirable effects. The mixing ratio is:
- 4 portions of blue powder ID9
- 3 portions of gray powder ID8.

③ **Translucent, sun-colored porcelain.** In certain cases this golden-yellow porcelain can be of great help, especially if a transparent T4 that is too gray is to be replaced. Usually, it is applied beneath the incisal layer,

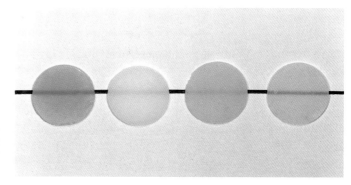

Fig 14-1 Four very useful original colors for daily practice. From left: translucent dark blue powder, opalescent white powder, mother-of-pearl-like incisal powder, translucent sun-colored powder (1-mm-thick samples).

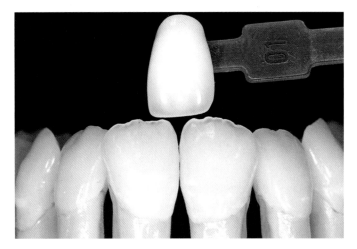

Fig 14-2 Note the dominant, slightly milky/cloudy, opalescent shade of these all-ceramic restorations. With these powders we can fabricate restorations that are brighter than the most brilliant color of the Ivoclar shade guide, without creating a restoration that is too opaque. Note the translucent, dark blue porcelain that was applied on the incisal edges in the background.

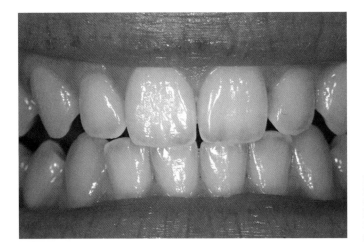

Fig 14-3 The blue translucency of the incisal edges of this young patient's teeth is conspicuous. In cases like this, the application of this translucent, dark blue porcelain is quite suitable.

thus light can circulate inside the layer and a gray tinge is avoided. We can use the same material as a translucent powder to define the "halo effect" at incisal edges (Fig 14-4). The mixing ratio of this translucent material is:
– 8 portions of neutral powder ID1
– 1 portion of orange powder ID5.
④ **Mother-of-pearl-like incisal porcelain.** This material is used most frequently. Thorough observation of natural teeth prove the use of this specific powder indispensable. This color corresponds to that of the internal surface of an oyster shell (Fig 14-5). The

porcelain is suitable as covering material for the incisal region, and its color is relatively common in teeth of middle-aged or older patients. This color, rarely found in ceramic powder kits, serves indisputably as an aid. Its fabrication, though, is considerably more difficult. The mixing ratio is as follows:
– 5 portions ID1 (neutral) + 1 portion ID2 (white)
– 3 portions ID8 (gray) + 2 portions ID7 (pink)
– 2 portions ID9 (blue).
Fabrication of these colors required numer-

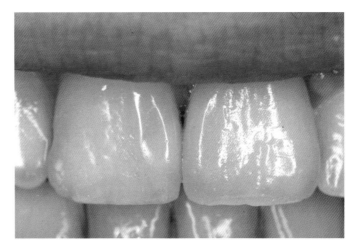

Fig 14-4 Metal ceramic crown on tooth 21. In order to create a "halo-effect" on the incisal edge, the translucent sun-colored porcelain was used. It was applied beneath the incisal layer so that light can freely circulate, but also for coverage of the gray tinge of the transparent porcelain T4.

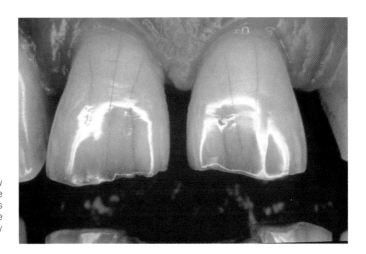

Fig 14-5 These natural teeth show the strong, mother-of-pearl-like shade of the incisal edge, which resembles the inner surface of an oyster. We have to use just this color to copy nature.

ous experiments (Fig 14-6). This facilitates evaluation and measuring whether it is equivalent to a ceramic layer that is predominantly used in most cases. In daily laboratory practice it is difficult to measure the correct quantity. Consequently, the material can neither be mixed instantly nor be stored.

If the mix is insufficiently homogeneous, it is likely to incorporate undesirable and unintended effects. My color palette, soon to be commercially available, will be a time saver.

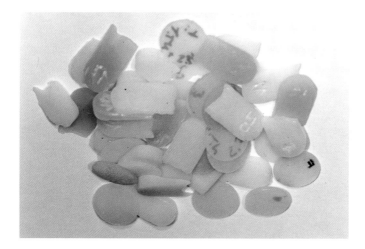

Fig 14-6 Much experimenting was done to accomplish a method of mixing for these powders.

15 Porcelain Inlays and Onlays

In 1886, a certain Mr Land introduced ceramic as a material for dental applications. The reason and the objective was the fabrication of a porcelain jacket crown that was fired onto a platinum foil matrix. During the following period of 15 years, porcelain inlays and onlays were subjects of somewhat enthusiastic acceptance that dwindled only after numerous cases of failure because of fracturing of the conventionally cemented (zinc phosphate) restorations and after Taggaret's invention of the lost-wax principle and casting technique.

The first inlays and onlays made of dental ceramic were fabricated as early as a hundred years ago. As a matter of fact, they preceded gold inlays but fell into oblivion for many decades. The development of precise refractory dies, the acid-etch technique used for enamel and porcelain, silanation of adhesive polymers, and the development of glass ionomer cement and new porcelain materials rehabilitated their clinical indication recently. These restorations now provide increased reliability and undeniable esthetic qualities.

In chapter 10 it is described how interesting sectioned teeth can be; collecting cross sections and photographs of teeth can serve as an aid in the attempt to imitate nature. These cross sections (they represent quite valuable material for instruction purposes) enabled the development of our layering technique, which uses more saturated colors in the center and less saturated ones at the surface. It can be used to fabricate both porcelain inlays and onlays. Their amazingly fine adaptation to natural teeth is a frequent cause for surprise, once they are cemented. The absence of metal creates unmatched esthetics and reduces the problem of metamerism. A whole new generation of reinforced porcelains with nonmetal or aluminum substructures has identical properties (see chapter 16, "Leucite-Reinforced Ceramic").

Here again it is necessary to work with numerous nuances and subtle colors in order to obtain satisfactory results. An inlay fabricated with one single dentin or incisal porcelain would appear totally lifeless after cementation. The interaction of shape and color becomes even more obvious regarding successful restorations of this kind (Fig 15-1).

General Criteria for Preparation of Ceramic Inlays and Onlays

In contrast to cavity preparations for gold inlays or onlays, the cavity preparation for porcelain inlays and onlays should not have axial walls that are too parallel (Fig 15-2). The friction exhibited by the inlay during try-in and cementation should be gentle; silanation and adhesive cementation provide sufficient retention. No bevel or chamfer is prepared at the cervical margins, but a groove is prepared instead with a round bur (Figs 15-3 to 15-6). That depression provides an extension of the corrodible enamel surface. No undercuts or 90° line angles at the cavity floor should exist (Fig 15-4).

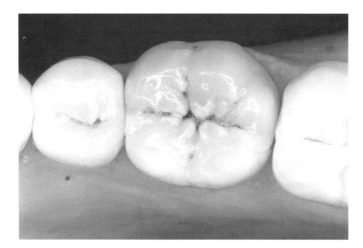

Fig 15-1 Two inlays on teeth 35 and 36. These inlays have been integrated in demineralized teeth of a skull. The objective of this study was not to fabricate monochromatic inlays and virtually restore the teeth the way they looked before. The main reason was to experiment with colors and shape in order to reconstruct a certain lifelike appearance.

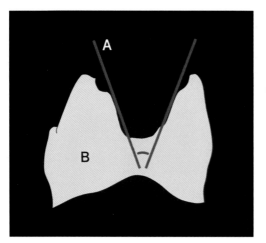

Fig 15-2 Preparation for a ceramic inlay. In contrast to gold inlays, where the axial walls must be as parallel as possible in order to provide for the necessary friction, the internal angles are much wider for ceramic inlays *(A)*. Friction is not the most important criterion, because we relate to adhesive techniques of cementation. Consequently, the preparation has to be modified.

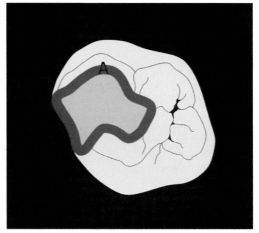

Fig 15-3 The margin formation should result in a semi-circular groove.

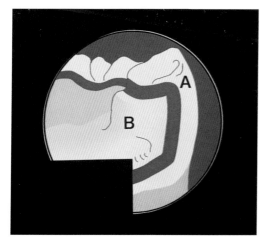

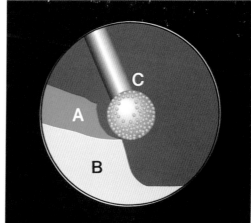

Fig 15-4 *(A)* A semicircular formation of the finish line. *(B)* The cavity floor should be rounded (ie, there should be no 90° angles).

Fig 15-5 The circumferential groove is best prepared with a round diamond *(C)*. This semicircular groove, which must be placed in the enamel *(A)*, increases the portion of the enamel surface that can be used for the etching procedure, thus also increasing adhesive retention. Furthermore, this preparation creates a satisfying transition between enamel and porcelain. The latter is particularly significant if a transparent porcelain will be used for the margins of the inlay.

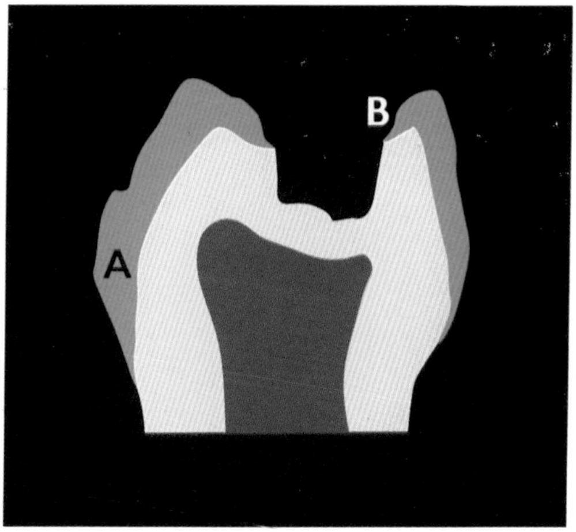

Fig 15-6 Cross section of a natural tooth. *(B)* Semicircular groove in the enamel layer *(A)*.

Preparing the Working Cast

After the impression is prepared in the usual manner and the working cast is fabricated using the Pindex system, we denude the margins if needed. A crayon is used to mark the finish line and the preparation is thinly coated twice with an ivory-colored die spacer (Fig 15-7). This primary cast serves for trial seatings of the inlays after the firing. An initial check reassesses the occlusal situation and contact points. This first cast is duplicated using the Cosmotech investment (GC International). I prefer this particular investment because of its precision and surface hardness. Only an investment material that is of absolute resistance can reproduce even the most minute detail of the finish line with the required accuracy. The refractory die is fabricated by means of the Pindex system using nonflammable pins by Optec (Fig 15-8). These pins will withstand the necessary firings unaltered and may be helpful for condensation, because they can act as a handle

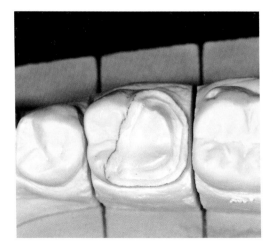

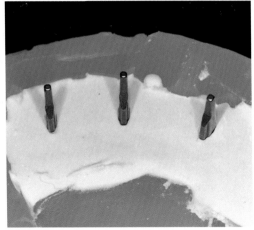

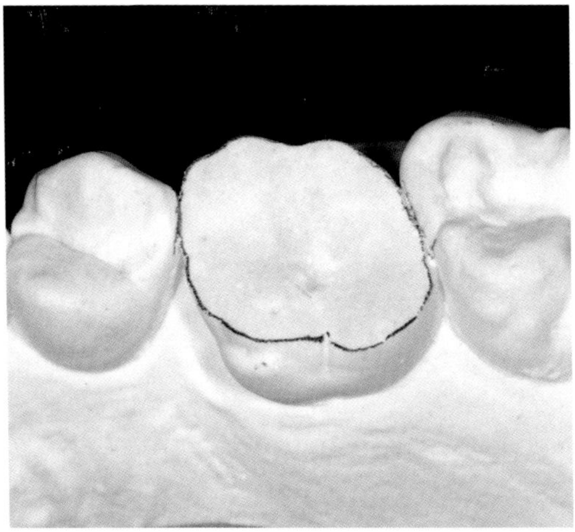

Fig 15-7 The finish line is marked with a crayon, and two coats of ivory-colored die spacer (Symphyse, Marseilles, France) are applied to the inlay cavity.

Fig 15-8 A refractory die model (Cosmotech, GC International) is cast by means of the Pindex system; nonflammable Optec pins are used.

Fig 15-9 A nonflammable pencil is used to mark the preparation margin of the inlay cavity on the die. A clearly visible finish line is very useful for successive firings.

when holding the die with tweezers. The refractory dies are separated and the finish line is trimmed if necessary.

The Cosmotech investment is white. Its color is an important detail, because it helps one to detect any mistake regarding color during the initial check after the firing. Investment material of a more intense color can influence the result and be the source of mistakes.

Thermal Processing of the Investment

Prior to **the first steps** of the procedure, the investment must undergo thermal treatment: a drying out period of 1 hour at 700°C should be allowed in a preheating oven. After all gases, particularly ammonium gases that are detrimental to the longevity of ceramic furnaces, have evaporated, the dies are removed from the oven and bench-cooled. The margin is then marked with a nonflammable pen; the

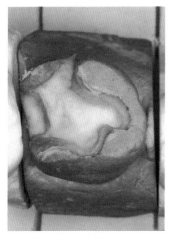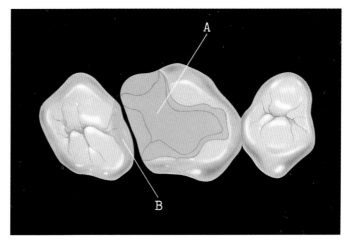

Figs 15-10 and 15-11 Wash bake. Transparent porcelain T4 is applied uniformly to the prepared portion of the die. The application should be extended beyond the finish line. The slurry is applied with maximum condensation. *(A)* Transparent porcelain T4; *(B)* transparent porcelain applied beyond the prepared portion.

marking is important especially with regard to the firings of the porcelain (Fig 15-9).

As a second step and completion of the thermal treatment, a firing sequence is performed. The die is placed in a ceramic furnace and vacuum fired. The initial temperature of 700°C is raised at a rate of 55°C per minute to a final 1,000°C, which should be maintained for 5 minutes. All inlay restorations fired on refractory dies require several firings, and it is impossible to fabricate porcelain inlays with just one bake. The attempt to fire too much bulk of porcelain at a time will inevitably result in detachment of the porcelain from the investment material. Therefore, the modeling procedure is preferably subdivided into several steps, and an extended firing cycle will generate better results.

Modeling of a Medium-Sized Inlay

First bake – wash bake. This significant step involves an attempt to produce a perfect bond between the porcelain and the investment material. Transparent porcelain T4 is applied to the prepared portion of the die, extending the covered area slightly over the margin. This thin layer is thought to reinforce the angles of the preparation and to supply a protective layer for the successive modeling of the porcelain, because ceramic tends to dry out rapidly (Figs 15-10 and 15-11).

The transparent layer should be as thin as possible, avoiding the application of too much porcelain to the internal line angles. In order to attain sufficient impregnation of the porcelain, you should condense maximally. The inlay must be dried prior to the firing for approximately 10 minutes according to a program similar to a bisque bake. After the firing the transparent layer should be virtually undetectable. Neither microfractures nor detachments of the porcelain should exist.

Second bake – firing the "intense" porcelain. During this bake the first layer of porcelain is applied. This must be the most saturated and most basic of all layers according to the layering technique. After moistening the die with distilled water, an orange porcelain is applied to the floor of the cavity in order to mimic the color of the pulp. This substance acts as an iridescent. The kind of orange to be selected depends on the patient's age. Orange-brown ID4 is suitable for

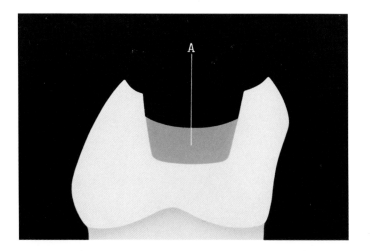

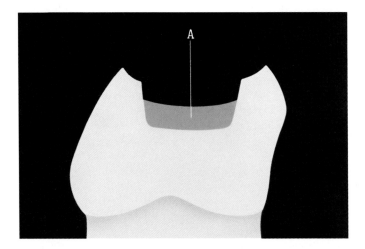

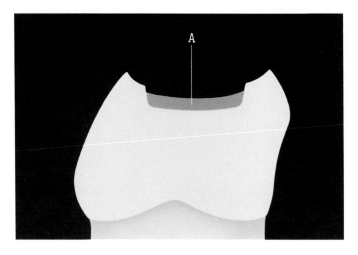

Figs 15-12 to 15-14 Prior to the firing of the "intense" porcelain, an intense orange is applied to the floor of the cavity (A). This material should mimic the color of the pulp and is the most saturated of the colors. The thickness of the layer depends on the depth of the cavity. The deeper the cavity, the more intense the orange, and vice versa.

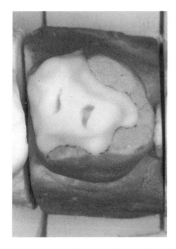 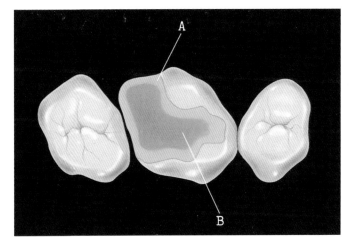

Figs 15-15 and 15-16 Firing of the "intense" porcelain. The intense orange (MY, Maverick kit), is applied to the floor of the cavity *(B)*. All margins are covered with transparent porcelain T4 without extending the application over the finish line *(A)*. This should create an optimal color transition from the ceramic to the enamel surface. In the center, the porcelain is cut through to the cavity floor. This cut effects a directed firing shrinkage from the center to the periphery, thus preventing a detachment of the material from the cavity walls.

all teeth of middle-aged or older patients, whereas "straw-colored," orange ID3 suits the teeth of younger patients. The amount of orange depends on cavity depth. The deeper the cavity the more intense the orange should be, and vice versa (Figs 15-12 to 15-14).

A masking dentin porcelain is applied to the upper region of the cavity (dentin-opaque by Ivoclar), and for completion, the transparent material T4 is used again thinly all along the margin to finish the build-up. However, this time the area of application is not extended over the cavosurface junction. The transparent porcelain T4 should create an optimal transition of colors from porcelain to the enamel surface (Figs 15-15 and 15-16).

Once the "intense" material is applied, the porcelain must be cut in a mesiodistal direction through to the floor of the cavity. This cut causes a controlled shrinkage from the center to the periphery during the bake, thus preventing a detachment of the porcelain from the cavity walls. Allow the die to dry for 10 minutes before the saturation bake. The firing cycle is identical to the wash bake.

Firing of the completed inlay. I build up

and bake medium-sized inlays at one time without an intermediate firing of the dentin porcelain. Occlusal surfaces are completed according to conventional procedures. The occlusal fissures are carved in the unbaked porcelain using a fissure-spatula, not a rotary instrument.

Utmost precision and care is exercised when modeling the inlay in slight supraocclusion in order to compensate for firing shrinkage (Figs 15-17 and 15-18). After firing, occlusal adjustment by selective grinding must be performed to conform to the individual situation.

By means of simultaneous firing of dentin, incisal, and transparent porcelains, the final contour of the inlay is virtually established. The articulator is used to detect and adjust premature contacts if necessary. The fissures are wider than usual, and often cusp ridges are not quite correct (Fig 15-19). Only one additional firing will be necessary.

Correction bake. This sequence of the firing procedure should complete the final contour, eliminate small defects, fill in voids and microfractures, and narrow the fissures. These corrections are made using incisal

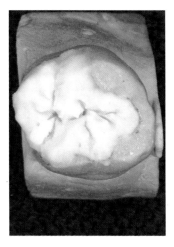
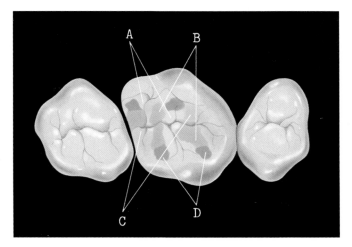

Figs 15-17 and 15-18 In just one single step, the modeling of the inlay is completed, including the use of numerous subtle color nuances. According to the principle of layering (ie, saturated color in the center and lightest color at the periphery), layer by layer of dentin porcelain is applied. With a spatula the fissures are carved into the still-plastic porcelain. *(A)* Glossy areas; *(B)* opalescent areas; *(C)* mother-of-pearl-like areas; *(D)* cusp summits colored with opaque dentin porcelain.

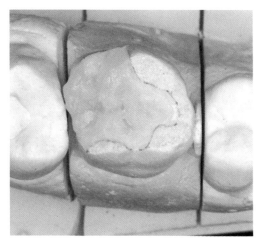

Fig 15-19 Inlay after the bake. Note: the orange color acts as an iridescent, and the minute color nuances are discernible. The margins of the inlay are precisely where the nonflammable pencil has marked the finish line.

porcelains that are vanilla-, mother-of-pearl-colored, opalescent, etc.

Thorough observation of a patient's natural teeth readily discloses these innumerable nuances. Even though these effects may be minute it would be a misconception to look at them as mere caricaturistic details. Equilibrium of these numerous nuances gives the inlay its natural appearance. Once again, the interaction of shape and color creates an "alive" impression (Figs 15-20 and 15-21).

Only after this firing sequence, when the occlusal fissures have been narrowed, is the grinding for occlusal adjustment performed. Now that the basic shape is accomplished, we can study the surface structure (Fig 15-22) and its macrogeography and microgeography using the polishing kit (see chapter 19, "Analysis of the Surface Structure – Polishing").

It helps to refer to photographs, extracted teeth, and working casts.

The inlay is then placed in the furnace to attain a low gloss. Provided there is sufficient space, minor corrections of the porcelain can be made. Then the inlay is vacuum fired. It is removed from the muffle and is polished to a high gloss (Fig 15-23) (see chapter 19).

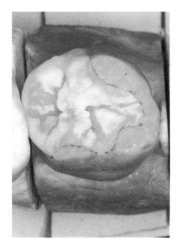 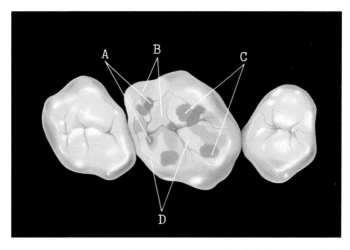

Figs 15-20 and 15-21 Correction bake. The correction bake completes the form, remedies deficiencies, and fills in possible cracks; it also serves to narrow the fissures. These corrections are made with incisal powders colored vanilla, mother-of-pearl, or opalescent. *(A)* Correction with opaque dentin powders; *(B)* opalescent corrections; *(C)* correction with dentin and transparent powder; *(D)* mother-of-pearl-colored corrections.

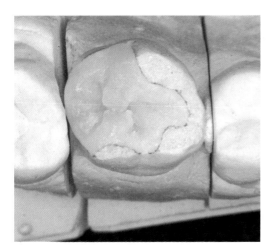 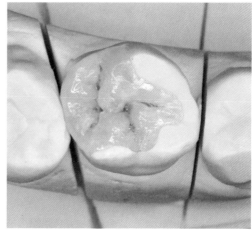

Fig 15-22 Inlay after the correction bake. The main interest is focused on the surface structure after the occlusal and functional relations have been inspected.

Fig 15-23 The finished ceramic inlay after polishing. This last step must be performed with the inlay seated on the die to prevent fractures.

Modeling of Smaller Inlays

Small inlays can be fabricated much quicker. The firing cycle is reduced, so that only two bakes will remain.

First bake – wash bake. The transparent porcelain T4 is used; this is inevitable if the modeling is to be performed on a refractory die. This very thin film of porcelain should be virtually invisible after the firing.

Second bake – firing the "intense" porcelain. An orange porcelain is applied to the center. It should mimic the color of the pulp. This material should be thicker in the center of the occlusal surface, thinning out to the margins. If we adhere to this recommendation, the orange material will be iridescent.

The transparent porcelain is applied at the margins, always bearing in mind not to extend over the finish line; once the inlay is cleaned of all investment, it may be difficult to correct these overcontoured areas. A masking dentin porcelain (opaque dentin) is applied to the most superficial portions of the cavity if necessary.

After the application of the "intense" material, the ceramic is cut in the center. This entire sequence of the procedure is identical to what has been described for medium-sized inlays.

Firing the completed inlay. The inlay is built up at one time. Again the layering technique is used – from saturated to less saturated porcelain powders, where a maximum of subtle vanilla-, mother-of-pearl-, and gold-colored ceramic powders is used. The inlay is more overcontoured than a metal ceramic restoration would be, the reason being a disproportion of the appropriate thickness inside the inlay cavity, and the fragility of the margins.

When the inlay is removed from the furnace, its occlusal anatomy should be almost established without any detachment of the porcelain. Small inlays usually show less dimensional discrepancy. The occlusion is inspected and the surface structure is established. Detected voids are filled in, and the floor of fissures may be characterized.

Glaze bake. Low gloss is required. The inlay is vacuum fired and the glaze bake is done concurrently with the correction bake. The low gloss should be preserved throughout the procedure. After the firing, polishing is performed with the restoration seated on the refractory die to avoid undue pressure exertion and protect the inlay from fracturing.

Modeling of Large Onlays

Very large onlays are not to be built up at one time. First only the dentin porcelain, which is thought to form the dentin core of the onlay, is applied. This first layer is fired (Figs 15-24 to 15-27). Very large restorations, which are built up on refractory dies to prevent the detachment of the porcelain from the investment, are fabricated in this manner. This method is recommendable for metal ceramic restorations of anterior teeth as well (see chapter 11, "Tricks to Make Porcelain Layering Easier"). It helps control the application of the dentin porcelain and also helps one evaluate the effects and characterizations deep within that layer. Even control of the occlusion is possible by means of selective grinding of the occlusal contacts.

A variety of porcelain powders is used to form the dentin core with the layering technique. The palette of colors, which we established earlier, already contains a number of nuanced colors. In more opalescent, yellowish, vanilla-colored, and mother-of-pearl-like regions, as well as for the cusp-cones an opaque dentin porcelain is applied (Fig 15-26). All of these small details underlying the transparent and incisal porcelain layers contribute to a more vital and natural appearance (Figs 15-28 and 15-29). The onlay is placed in the furnace for 9 minutes to be dried, and a conventional dentin bake is carried out.

After the firing, the surface must be ground to a matte finish to facilitate and improve bonding to the successively applied transparent and incisal porcelains. With the application of additional effects and the incisal

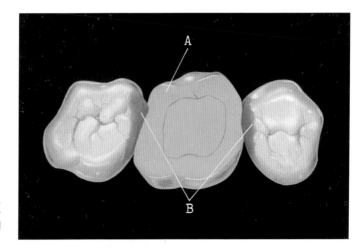

Fig 15-24 Wash bake of a large-sized onlay. *(A)* Transparent powder T4; *(B)* transparent powder extended over the cavity margins.

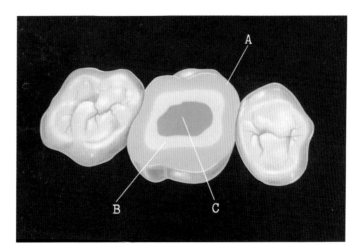

Fig 15-25 Firing of the "intense" porcelain. The ceramic material must be cut in the center to control shrinkage. An opaque dentin *(B)* is applied to the highest points of the cavity. The margins receive a layer of transparent porcelain *(A)*. *(C)* Intense orange MY.

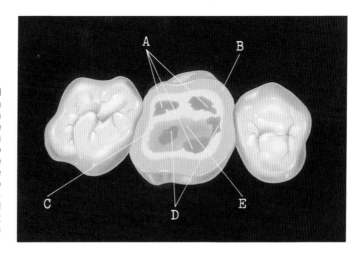

Fig 15-26 Very large onlays should preferably be modeled only with dentin and effect porcelain, which represent the dentin core of the onlay. Very large restorations, which are built up on refractory dies to prevent the detachment of the porcelain from the investment, are fabricated in this manner. *(A)* Cusp summit with opaque dentin; *(B)* transparent margins; *(C)* slightly saturated dentin powder; *(D)* opalescent region; *(E)* more saturated dentin powder in the center.

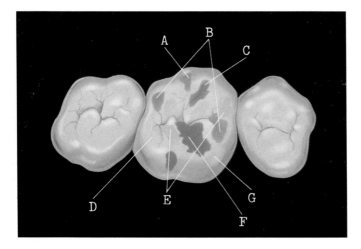

Fig 15-27 Modeling of the onlay is completed with the application of the incisal and effect powders. The colors we used are from the IPS Classic and Maverick kit by Ivoclar. *(A)* Intense orange MY; *(B)* opalescent area 101 + T4; *(C)* cusp summits of opaque dentin powder; *(D)* incisal porcelain of varying brilliance; *(E)* vanilla-colored areas B-LB5; *(F)* gray-brown powder B-DB3; *(G)* yellow areas BY3.

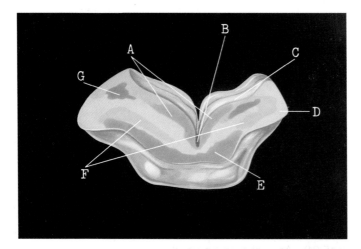

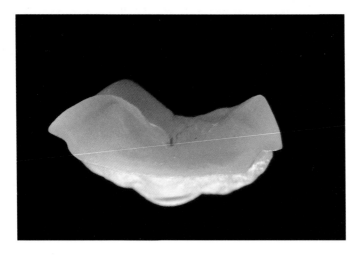

Figs 15-28 and 15-29 Cross section of an onlay in order to illustrate the layering technique and the principle of saturated colors in the center and decreasing saturation toward the periphery. Note the enamel superimposed on the transparent porcelain. This is a very useful example to demonstrate all the various characterizations as well as the interplay of shape and color. *(A)* Opalescent areas ID2 + D1C; *(B)* brown metal oxide 107; *(C)* incisal powder S1; *(D)* transparent margins T4; *(E)* orange dentin powder M-HY; *(F)* dentin powder 1C; *(G)* dentin powder 1C + vanilla-colored powder.

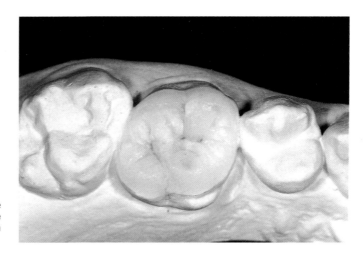

Fig 15-30 Onlay after the glaze bake: low gloss achieved. Now the onlay can be polished to a high gloss.

porcelain, the modeling is completed (Fig 15-27). At the end of the entire procedure, the onlay is treated in the same manner as described for small and medium-sized inlays (Fig 15-30).

Removal of the Investment

Removal of the investment is a difficult but important step. In order to guard against fracturing, the inlay, which is seated on the refractory die, is invested in silicone compound; the marginal region is covered (Fig 15-31). As soon as the compound has set, the investment can be removed with an air abrasion unit, abrasive glass beads, and the pressure of 3 bar. Thus, the fragile margins as well as the whole restoration will be protected. The underside of the onlay has a gentle, matte gloss, and even the finest detail at the margins will be preserved after air abrasion because of the silicone (Fig 15-32).

Inspection of the marginal fit. The use of the investment material (Cosmotech, GC International) facilitates precise dental ceramic restorations. Possible overcontouring can be corrected with abrasive stones. This correction is made easier if the margins have been marked with a special nonflammable pen.

Gold inlays must exhibit strong friction; this is not so with ceramic inlays, because they attain a tight seal by silanation and adhesive cementation. Too much friction would incorporate an additional risk at try-in. If you encounter a case of problematic friction that is difficult to localize, use a blue friction paste included in the Empress (Ivoclar) kit. The paste must cover the underside of the inlay. Thus, after trial seating of the restoration, the areas of tightness are readily discernible and can be reduced. For this task, a dissecting microscope with considerable magnification should be used.

Occlusal conditions cannot be inspected during trial seatings of ceramic inlays and onlays; this is done after cementation (Fig 15-33). To do so at an earlier stage may put the restoration at risk.

After the last inspection of the marginal fit and occlusion in the articulator, the inlay is completed. Now the etching must be done. An etching gel is used that contains hydrofluoric and sulphuric acid (Symphyse, Marseilles, France). The gel is applied to the underside of the inlay and allowed to stand for 3 minutes. Accidental application to the occlusal surface must be avoided by all means. The inlay is rinsed thoroughly with a strong spray to remove the gel. It is placed on

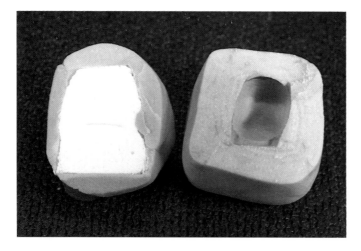

Fig 15-31 Inlay on the refractory die, invested in a silicone compound. As soon as the silicone compound has set, the investment material is removed with an air abrasion unit without endangering the margin of the restoration or the risk of fracture. Air abrasion is performed with glass beads and 3 bar of pressure. The silicone is later removed with a scalpel.

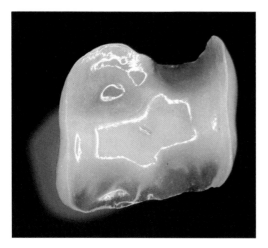

Fig 15-32 Underside of a ceramic onlay. Note the orange-colored material mimicking the color of the pulp and the margins of transparent powder.

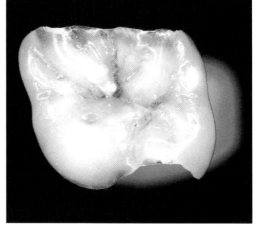

Fig 15-33 The occlusal view reveals all subtleties of characterization, which provide an "alive" appearance.

a nonflammable cotton-wool pad and placed in the furnace for 15 minutes at 550°C. After this treatment, which removes all acid residue, the inlay is ready for adhesive cementation.

The fabrication of ceramic inlays is quite an exciting procedure. The dental technician must precisely follow the procedures in order to create a successful inlay (Figs 15-34 to 15-39). The single step of the procedure is not particularly time consuming, but multiple firings are required. This high-quality integration in the patient's mouth is the sum of important parameters: the interaction of color and shape, good teamwork, and a mutual understanding between dentist and dental technician.

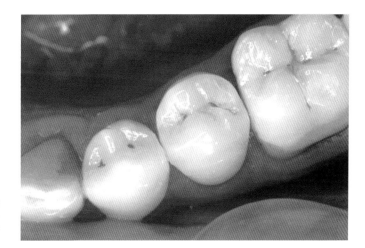

Fig 15-34 Porcelain onlay on tooth 35. Note the delicate fissures. (Courtesy of Dr Bernard Touati, Paris, France.)

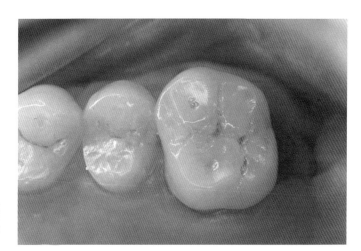

Fig 15-35 Porcelain onlay on tooth 26. Very satisfying mimicry with natural teeth. (Courtesy of Dr Bernard Touati, Paris, France.)

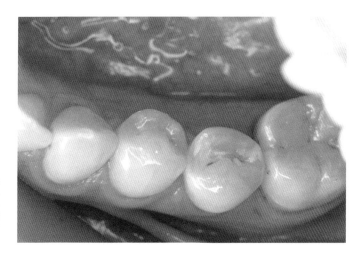

Fig 15-36 Porcelain onlay on tooth 35. Note the opalescent and vanilla-colored areas. Good color adaptation with regard to the enamel of the natural teeth. (Courtesy of Dr Bernard Touati, Paris, France.)

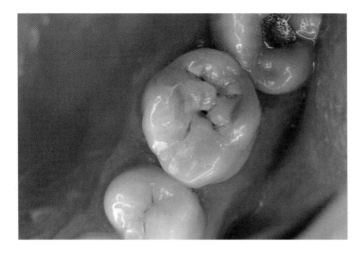

Fig 15-37 Porcelain inlay on tooth 16. This poor color is a result of the application of too strong "intense" colors beneath the incisal layers. If it is difficult to evaluate the influence of the underlying colors, the application of transparent powders at the margins is not recommended.

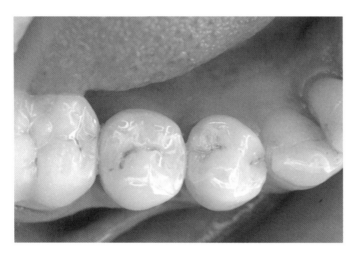

Fig 15-38 Porcelain inlays on teeth 44 and 45, immediately after adhesive cementation. The margins are still visible.

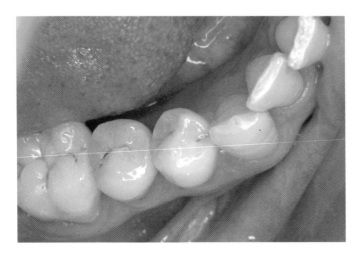

Fig 15-39 After the final polishing inside the patient's mouth, the conspicuous margins become indiscernible. The color transitions are very satisfactory. This work is an apt example of successful teamwork and mutual understanding between dentist and dental technician.

Natural-Appearing Fissures

Restorations with fissures that strongly re-semble wide and straight canals are a famil-iar sight. They do not exhibit the slightest sim-ilarity to natural occlusal fissures. To remedy this deficiency, esthetic and functional aspects must be coupled. If we study natural teeth (which should always be at hand), certain irregularities can be observed. The fissures are not arranged in a straight-line pattern; they are curvy and go up and down, not unlike a sine curve (Fig 15-40). Standard restorations are all too often recognized as "prostheses"; they are too regular in form, color, and fissures. Once integrated in the mouth, the result can be rather disappoint-ing. Therefore, we must struggle against rigid methods that produce stereotyped restora-tions. We must try to approach nature as closely as possible, because nature has pur-posefully created irregularities in symmetry.

A small, flat-edged spatula which is bent at its rounded end is the instrument for model-ing fissures in porcelain. Playful use of this spatula and the creamy porcelain mix creates occlusal surfaces that look "alive." We pick into the fossae of the main fissures, come back to the surface, go down to the floor of the fissure again, and finally smooth the fissure at its summit. This pattern of move-ments forms small enamel ridges that create vitality (Figs 15-41 to 15-43). The acute point can be used to narrow the fissures at this stage (Fig 15-44). Meanwhile, occlusal con-cepts must not be neglected; they are of first priority. It is not time-consuming to create occlusal surfaces that way; it is significant, though, to maintain moisture and plasticity so that the porcelain is not prone to cracking. After the modeling procedure, the somewhat dry porcelain is brushed with a flexible brush (particularly the occlusal surface) in the direc-tion of the fissures (Fig 15-45).

During the first bake the porcelain shrinks; small portions will shift dimensionally. The fissures will look natural thereafter. In par-ticular, the floor of the fissures will be distinctly visible without the use of even the smallest

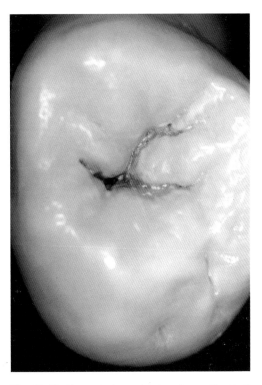

Fig 15-40 If we study occlusal surfaces of natural teeth, we can observe that fissures are not arranged in a straight-line pattern. On the contrary, they are curvy and go up and down, not unlike a sine curve. This is caused by the ridges of the two cusps.

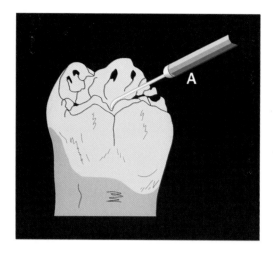

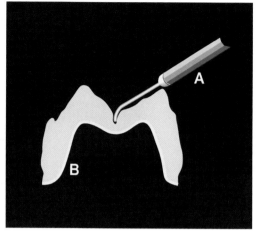

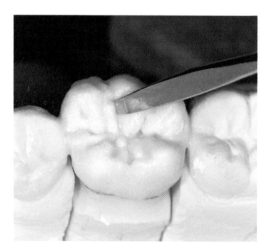

Fig 15-41 Spatula for the formation of natural-looking fissures *(A)*. It is a small, flat-edged spatula that is bent at its rounded end. With this spatula, (ie, its rounded end), we pick into the fossae and preform the shape of cusps out of the porcelain.

Fig 15-42 Cross section of a metal ceramic crown *(B)*. The spatula is used to fabricate natural-looking fissures.

Fig 15-43 The fissure is formed in the ceramic slurry. Note the degree of moisture on the material.

Fig 15-44 The acute point of the modeling brush is suitable for narrowing the fissures and creating small enamel ridges.

Fig 15-45 When the modeling is finished, the occlusal surface is smoothed with a very flexible brush, always working parallel to the fissure direction. At this stage it is important that the porcelain be somewhat dried.

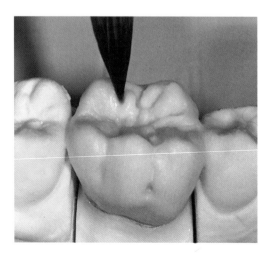

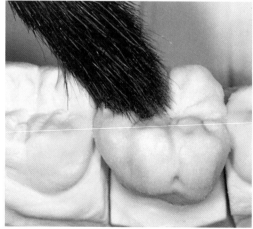

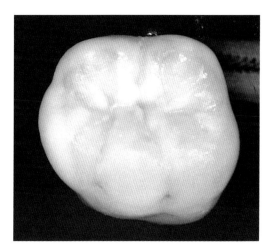

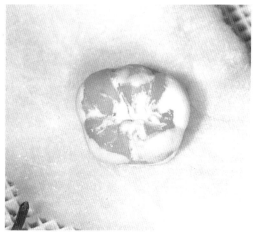

Fig 15-46　During the second firing the fissures can be narrowed with the point of a modeling brush. To mix the powder we use a high-viscosity liquid (glazing liquid). This should prevent the correction porcelain from drying out prematurely.

Fig 15-47　The crown is placed on a nonflammable cotton-wool pad. We allow an extended drying period (4 minutes) in order to completely remove the high-viscosity liquid.

grinder. Thus, we obtain natural-looking fissures without the need to use rotary instruments.

During the second bake, the fissures can be narrowed with the point of a modeling brush (Figs 15-46 and 15-47).

As we have seen, fissures of ceramic restorations can look natural (Figs 15-48 to 15-53). The use of rotary instruments should be strictly avoided.

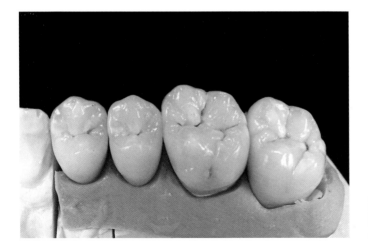

Fig 15-48 Metal ceramic crowns. Note the natural-looking fissures. The interplay of shape and color is clearly visible.

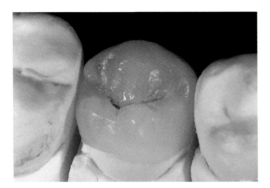 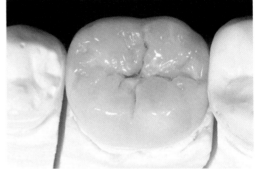

Figs 15-49 and 15-50 Porcelain onlays. The natural-looking fissures are delicate.

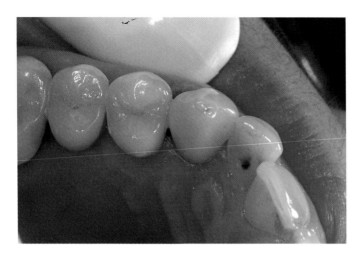

Fig 15-51 Empress ceramic restorations on teeth 13, 14, and 15. (Courtesy of Dr Michel Canazzi, Caderousse, France.)

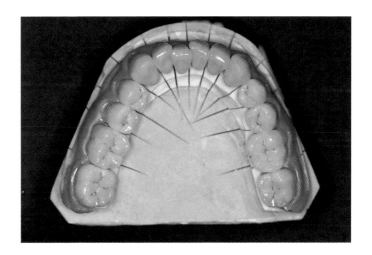

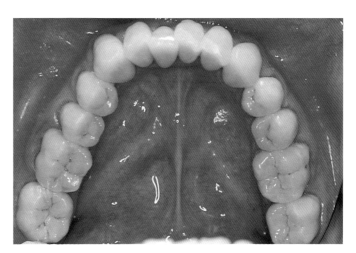

Figs 15-52 and 15-53 Fourteen metal ceramic crowns in situ. (Courtesy of Dr Luc Portalier, Aix-en-Provence, France.)

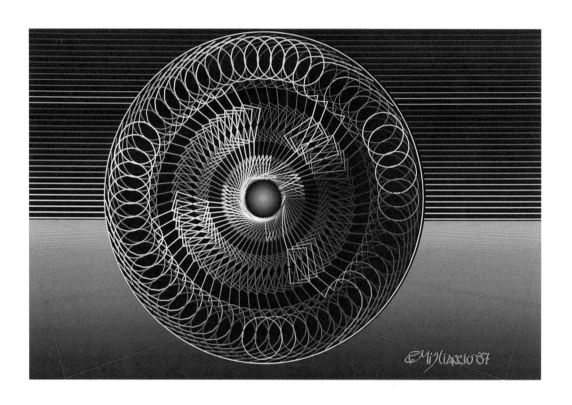

16 Leucite-Reinforced Ceramic

Currently, there are some exciting new developments in our profession; the properties of materials and the applied techniques are constantly improving. New nonmetal porcelains, which are reinforced with leucite, possess incomparable esthetic qualities. The absence of metal, or aluminum substructures eliminates even the slightest hint of reflection within the restoration. Light can circulate inside and even penetrate the restoration, which is very similar to what happens inside a natural tooth. Furthermore, the phenomenon of metamerism, well known in the field of metal ceramics, will be reduced.

All these characteristics contribute to the success of porcelain restorations and help to make the ceramist's task easier. These new porcelains may also help provide a satisfying prosthodontic result for patients who demand a highly esthetic restoration.

Empress System (Ivoclar). In June 1990, a new system was introduced to our laboratory: IPS Empress by Ivoclar. This unique system is particularly satisfying because of its simple and uncomplicated method of processing. There is no need to alter established laboratory procedures, because this new system proves very similar to the lost-wax technique. It is also possible to make use of the layering technique. But most of all, we can adhere to the principle to begin the build-up with a colored ceramic core, thus influencing the color of a restoration from the inside (see chapter 10, "Processing and Natural Layering of Metal Ceramic").

In addition, a significant advantage lies in the fact that there is no need to fabricate and work with a refractory die while modeling the

restoration (the necessary extended drying cycles would consume time, because we could not afford to leave the furnace). Furthermore, there is no risk of warpage, which often occurs when working with refractory die models, where application of proximal contacts or correction of color and occlusion requires reinvestment for several successive firings.

IPS Empress: A New Technology in Dental Ceramics

History

The Greek word "keramos" means pottery or "fired matter." Humankind has known about fire for 400,000 years, and the first specimens of "fired matter" are dated from 23,000 BC. From the first simple objects made of soil and clay, the use of "fired matter" changed and developed with experience, from the Stone Age to space technology and to the high technology of the twentieth century.

The French chemist Duchateau is said to have first used porcelain as a dental material in 1776. The Parisian dentist Dubois de Chemant developed this idea further, and in 1788 the first artificial teeth made of porcelain were produced. At the beginning of this century the porcelain "jacket" crown as a prosthodontic restoration for severely damaged teeth was introduced by C.H. Land. This kind of restoration was widely used until the advent of porcelain-fused-to-metal crowns in the 1960s.

Thanks to new technologies and materials, the all-ceramic crown was revived in the early 1980s, because metal ceramic crowns did not measure up to increased esthetic demands.

The forerunner of these nonmetal ceramic crowns may well have been the Dicor and Cerestore Systems. The potential for esthetic restorations using these systems initiated the introduction of other ceramic systems with which crowns, inlays, and veneers could be fabricated on refractory dies; the systems were marketed under names such as Fortune, Hi-Ceram, Mirage, and Optec.

The Achilles' heel of ceramic materials is brittleness and, consequently, a tendency to fracture. It was assumed that atomic bonds would provide adequate strength. However, this expectation cannot be fulfilled in practice, because of the phenomenon of microscopic surface defects, which propagate under stress and ultimately lead to gross fractures.

One of the current developments for decreasing the tendency to fracture is the incorporation of fibers. However, their fabrication and application in the field of dental ceramics are still in the initial stage.

Another approach for minimizing the propagation of microfractures and thus improving porcelain strength is glass ceramics. Characteristic for this material is the controlled crystallization of glass. The process forms a two-phase crystalline material with a relatively high proportion of a vitreous matrix. Because of nucleus formation and crystal growth, microcrystals are formed throughout the entire glass matrix if the correct temperature is maintained. These nuclei are either a latent function within the glass or intentionally introduced and finely dispersed.

The heterogeneous structure of the material and/or the generation of compressive stress at the phase interfaces results in a considerable increase of strength and decrease of tendency to fracture.

Thanks to these major advantages of the new technology, a large variety of applications has been created for vitreous materials, including dental technology.

The application of glass ceramic as a dental material was attempted in 1968 by MacCulloch. However, it took 20 more years until the companies of Corning and Dentsply were able to bring the first commercially available product on the market. The introduction of "castable" ceramic was undoubtedly a significant step in the history of dental ceramic. It created remarkable interest among experts, which was reflected in the large number of publications. At about the same time, researchers at the University of Zürich tried to develop heat-pressed ceramic as a prosthodontic material, which was later marketed by Ivoclar. Investigations in literature (a prerequisite for patent registration) later revealed that this idea had been published as early as 1936.

The systematic development of a specific type of glass ceramic not only helped accomplish objectives like improvement of strength and esthetics, it also perfected a system with a simplified method of fabrication. A 3-year clinical trial phase confirmed expectations. The following pages present the materials and the applied method.

The Material

General View

A colorless base material that exhibits sufficient transparency and minimum porosity is necessary to produce an all-ceramic restoration. Furthermore, the material should have the following properties:
- Simple processing
- Exact duplication of the wax models and high stability of form during further firing cycles (eg, staining, glazing)
- Adequate strength under consideration of a safety margin to withstand functional loading by masticatory forces
- Chemical stability under intraoral conditions

Composition

Porcelain that meets the requirements mentioned above is manufactured from two basic glass melts labeled Ti^{4+}. The ceramic system comprises the following materials:
- Pressed ceramic for the staining
- Pressed ceramic for the layering technique
- Surface stains
- Corrective porcelain
- Layer ceramic
- Glazing powder

The different materials are manufactured from the basic glass or mixtures of the glass with additives such as color pigments, fluorescent substances, or elements to achieve a higher melting point (see the following table).

The basic glass is melted in a continuous crucible furnace at 1,450°C. After the first firing and to ensure homogeneity, the melt is quenched, dried, ground, and remelted. By means of a tempering process (temperature/time), the amorphous glass is transformed into glass ceramic. Parameters of this process can be varied, thus optimizing the material characteristics and ensuring that they comply with the requirements of the system components.

Composition of the basic glass (wt/%)

Oxide	Melt 1	Melt 2
SiO_2	63.0	61.0
Al_2O_3	17.7	14.3
K_2O	11.2	10.1
Na_2O	4.6	8.0
B_2O_3	0.6	0.6
CeO_2	0.4	0.9
CaO	1.6	3.3
BaO	0.7	1.5
TiO_2	0.2	0.3

Microstructure

The characteristic features of a ceramic material are specified in particular by its structure, both at the atomic level and at the microscopic level.

At the atomic level, ceramic material is characterized by two types of bonds: ionic and covalent. The ionic bond is characterized by an exchange of electrons. The atom that gives up an electron to a neighboring atom is positively charged, whereas the other atom receiving the electron consequently assumes a negative charge. Opposite charges attract, and the atoms are bound to one another. With the covalent bond, the electrons (one or more than one) are shared by neighboring atoms (Figs 16-1 and 16-2).

Although the electrostatic attraction between neighboring atoms is reduced compared to the ionic bond, covalent bonds demonstrate an atomic orientation that limits the movement of atoms. The hardest known material, the diamond, consists of carbon atoms in a covalent bond.

Regardless of the type of bond, the atoms are able to form groups. Any such configuration that is a regular pattern throughout the body of the material is referred to as a crystal. The identical combination of atoms can form

143

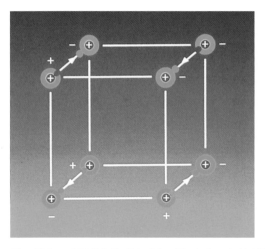 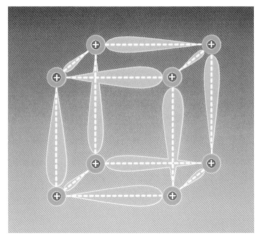

Figs 16-1 and 16-2 *(left)* Principle of ionic bond. *(right)* Principle of covalent bond.

either an amorphous or a crystalline structure. This depends on whether the atoms have sufficient time for orientation during the formation process. If, for instance, silicon dioxide is fused and then cooled slowly, the SiO_2 molecules form a macroscopic lattice of cristobalite crystals. If the same material is cooled rapidly, allowing the molecules no time for orientation, then the product is an amorphous substance: glass.

The abundance of atomic structures as well as the numerous possibilities of combining or exchanging chemical elements provide a virtually unlimited variety of ceramic substances, all of radically different properties. The atomic structure of porcelain supplies the material with high chemical resistance to intraoral conditions. The strength of the atomic bond is also responsible for a high fusing point, great hardness, and strength.

Unfortunately, this stability of bonds simultaneously prevents a sliding movement of the atoms within the structure. For that reason, the material cannot be deformed by external forces at room temperature. Consequently, to a certain limit porcelain has extraordinary dimensional stability under loading; beyond that limit, the linkage collapses suddenly and the material fractures.

This brittleness is the cause for an additional characteristic: ceramic material can bear compressive stress rather than tensile stress or shearing forces. Compressive loads tend to close developing microfractures whereas tensile or shearing loads will widen them.

Ceramic material would be much more resistant if defects created during fabrication or by mechanical strain could be avoided. Stress is concentrated particularly upon these defects. Because porcelain does not provide sufficient elasticity to compensate for such stress, the critical limit mentioned before is easily exceeded. Consequently, the ceramic breaks (Figs 16-3 and 16-4).

In order to increase the strength of vitreous objects, we can apply methods that reduce the effects of microfractures and defects in the surface of the material. One of these methods is the "hardening" of glass. The material is heated to the temperature of transformation and then cooled rapidly by blowing cold air over the surface. During this process the surface of the glass cools down quickly while the layer beneath contracts further. Inevitably, the result is compressive stress at the surface and tensile stress within the object. The tensile stress within the inferior layer

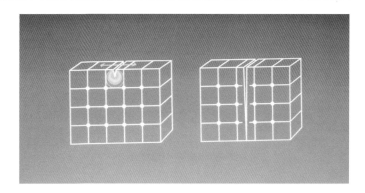

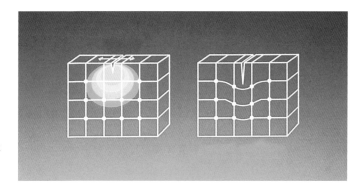

Figs 16-3 and 16-4 *(above)* Crack propagation in brittle materials. *(below)* Crack propagation in plastic, elastic, and ductile materials.

compensates the surface stress. This pressure effect closes the microfractures in the glass, thus preventing their propagation. The danger of fracture rises only when the tensile component outweighs the compressive one (Fig 16-5). During the glaze bake, compressive stress may develop in the porcelain. This happens when the coefficient of thermal expansion of the glazing material is smaller than that of the underlying porcelain.

The concept of creating compressive stress can be transferred to the microscopic field. If crystals are produced that possess higher thermal expansion than the surrounding glass matrix, the matrix is subjected to compressive stress at the periphery of these crystals. The larger the difference of expansion between the glass and the crystalline phase, the better the strength. This is the principle of material reinforcement that the Empress system capitalizes on.

Controlled Crystallization: Theoretic Fundamentals

Crystallization was once one of the most undesirable phenomena in the production of glass. Later it was appreciated as a benefit with regard to industrial use: the new glass ceramics (or vitro ceramics) were developed.

The accidentally occurring crystallization (ie, the failures that appeared during glass manufacture) demonstrated a wide variety of different sizes of crystals. In homogeneous glass, a condition is sometimes found where a critical size of the nuclei is exceeded and a nucleus grows to uncontrollable size. The controlled crystallization is distinguished from the sporadic crystal growth by the following criteria:

145

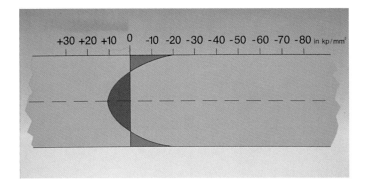

+30 +20 +10 0 -10 -20 -30 -40 -50 -60 -70 -80 in kp/mm²

Fig 16-5 Inherent stress distribution within "hardened" glass.

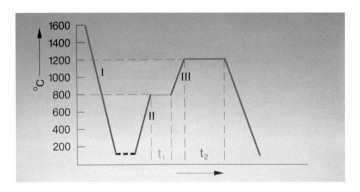

Fig 16-6 Formation of glass ceramic, according to Stookey (*green* = crystallization temperature; *yellow* = nucleation temperature). *I* = working phase, *II* = nucleation, *III* = crystallization.

- Nucleus formation rate is high and regular throughout the entire glass matrix
- Crystals are small and of uniform size (only a few micrometers)

Characteristic for glass ceramic is the presence of small concentrations of crystallization or mineralization nuclei (eg, fluorides, phosphates, titandioxides).

The primary process of any controlled crystallization within the glass is the separation of microphases during the cooling period of the melt. The progression of such a process has been thoroughly investigated and described by W. Vogel. Typical steps in the transformation of glass into glass ceramic (Fig 16-6) are:

1. Glass is melted, ground, and cooled down.
2. The object is heated to the temperature T_1 (temperature of nucleus formation); at temperature T_1 over time t_1, the nuclei are formed.
3. After completion of t_1, the temperature is advanced further to level T_2 (crystallization temperature). At temperature T_2, crystallization occurs over time t_2, and glass is transformed into glass ceramic.

Mere visual investigation shows distinct differences between the glass samples and the tempered glass. The samples made of glass are transparent, whereas the ones made of tempered glass are cloudy.

Structure Analysis

In the field of ceramics, ceramography (which is analogous to the metallographic methodology) is used to analyze microscopic structure.

In order to permit differentiation of the crystal phases, selective etching is performed. Generally 0.1% to 0.5% hydrofluoric acid (HF) is used. By means of controlled variation of acid concentration and/or the etching time, the crystalline phases and their microstructure can be investigated.

Because the dimension of the crystals is in the order of micrometers and our major interest is the microstructure, scanning electron microscopy is used. The scanning procedure reveals that untempered glass has no structure. Tempered basic glass, on the other hand, shows a specific microstructure after etching (0.5% HF, for 1 minute):

● Crystals with a lamellar microstructure are found embedded in an amorphous matrix.

Based on the composition of glass, which consists mainly of $SiO_2 - Al_2O_3 - K_2O$, the formation of a low leucite is very likely ($K_2O - Al_2O_3 - 4\ SiO_2$). The microstructure found in the tempered glass is very similar to the low leucite crystals discovered by Barreiro. Small quantities of additives ($< 5\%$) mixed to the basic glass result in pressed ceramic. The microstructure has changed; the crystallites are apparently smaller and more densely dispersed.

Microfractures within the crystals are immediately apparent. This phenomenon is explained not only by a different coefficient of thermal expansion between the leucite and the matrix glass but even moreso by contraction. This contraction occurs concurrent to a phase change from high leucite to low leucite during the cooling process.

Bowen described that the propagation of microfractures in a material is prevented when the tip of a crack enters a microfracture. Both ends of a microfracture are then rounded and smoothed as a result of the successive firing. Such microfractures are created purposefully and intentionally to achieve increased fracture resistance in ceramic material.

Crystal Identification by Radiographic Analysis

Radiographic methods can aid in identifying minerals or mineral components based on their microstructure. Using a Guinier-IV-camera (made by Nonius, Delft) and Cu-Kδ-radiation it was possible to analyze an x-ray diffraction spectrum of a powder that was obtained from two melts of the basic ceramic. The qualitative determination of the crystalline phases was performed by comparing all d-values to the data of the ASTM card index.

The x-ray-diffraction spectra for the basic glass show a structure that is x-ray amorphous. The tempered glass, in contrast, shows an x-ray spectrum of a low leucite if it is compared to the ASTM card index (Fig 16-7). These tests on the coefficient of thermal expansion provide further indication for the leucite crystal formation. While the coefficient of basic glass is 10 μm/(m · $^\circ$K), it is 17 μm/(m · $^\circ$K) for tempered glass (Fig 16-8). For leucite a value of 20 μm/(m · $^\circ$K) is mentioned. This could explain the increased coefficient of thermal expansion for the formation of leucite.

Strength

As previously described, prevention of crack propagation plays a central role for the strength of porcelain. A homogeneous, monolithic material fails to inhibit crack propagation. This cannot be prevented and will result in spontaneous fracturing. In a heterogeneous substance, different phases can prevent crack formation. The result is an increased resistance to fracture.

A multiple-phase, heterogeneous porcelain exhibits anisotropic stress after cooling down (Fig 16-9). On the one hand, leucite crystals are subject to stronger contraction after cooling down compared to the glass matrix because of higher thermal expansion. On the other hand, the transformation from a cubical

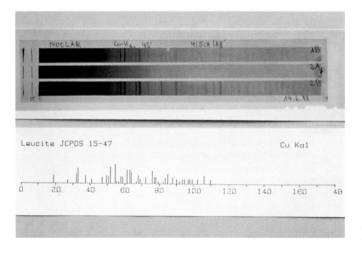

Fig 16-7 X-ray diffraction spectra. *2A* = amorphous basic glass; *1B*, *2B* = tempered glass.

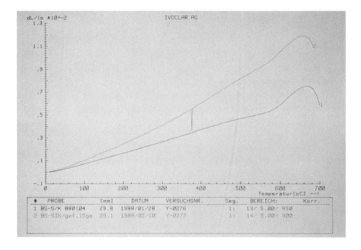

Fig 16-8 TEC-diagram: basic glass *(red)*, tempered glass *(green)*.

high leucite to a tetragonal low leucite during this thermal contraction leads to a volume reduction in the order of 1.2%. During this cooling period the two phases (leucite crystals and glass matrix) remain in intimate contact. As the material solidifies, tangential compressive stress in the glass matrix and radial tensile stress in the leucite develop. These stresses are initially balanced.

The final phase of contraction leads to crack formation within the leucite, because tensile stress wins out over tensile strength. This causes a simultaneous partial disconnection (separation) of glass matrix and leucite crystals. The initial balance between the forces changes to a dominance of the compressive portion (Fig 16-10). The compressive strength of the glass matrix is sufficiently high to "freeze" compressive stress at the phase interface. According to this model, a latently existing compressive stress can decrease the spontaneous formation of microfractures. Furthermore, a dispersive structure at the phase interface leads to a diversion of

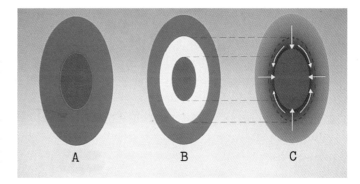

Fig 16-9 Radial and tangential stress produced by different TEC of glass and leucite. *(A)* Glass *(green)* and leucite *(red)* in heated plastic condition. *(B)* Contraction of glass and leucite during cooling period without adhesion. *(C)* Cooling with adhesion produces tangential compressive stress in the glass and radial tensile stress in the leucite. (According to Prasad, et al; α leucite $>$ α glass.

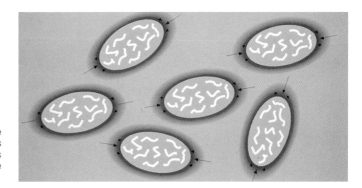

Fig 16-10 Tangential compressive stress – radial tensile stress. Stress condition in completed Empress restoration. The microfractures in the leucite "release" the tensile stress.

microfractures, thus diminishing the fracture energy.

Latently present microfractures with rounded tips can limit or even prevent crack propagation.

This technique can be seen as the ingenious and ancient concept of architectural arch construction transferred into microscopic dimensions and thereby realized a structurally reinforced dental porcelain. The compressive forces are substantially stronger than the gravitational forces of the bricks. These conditions secure great stability (Fig 16-11). Another example is modern reinforced concrete, where elements of steel create compressive stress within the concrete. By using the tensile strength of steel and the compressive strength of concrete combined, both of superior quality, constructions can be built that withstand enormous strain.

(This section contributed by *Gerhard Beham,* chemist, department for research and development, Ivoclar Corp.)

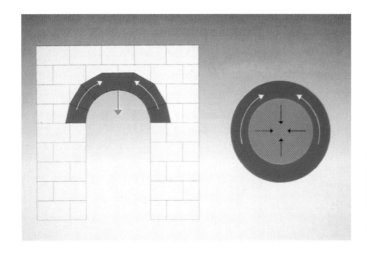

Fig 16-11 Compressive stress at the phase interface of the glass matrix (*green* = radial tensile stress) and leucite crystals (*red* = tangential compression) is comparable with the construction principle of an arch. According to Mackert; α leucite > α glass.

Working Procedures

The Muffle

Crowns, inlays, and veneers are all modeled in wax (Fig 16-12). Similar to the technique of metal casting, the wax modeling must be invested in a specific refractory investment material (Fig 16-13). A specially designed muffle system is required for the investment of the wax-up and the placement of the ceramic ingots.

The completed wax-up is sprued and safely attached to the cylindrical crucible former. A prefabricated paper investment ring is placed on the base of the special crucible former. A supplied stabilizing ring is then attached to the top of the construction. Thus, a cylindric form is created that is filled with the investment.

When the material has hardened, the setting expansion will later facilitate devesting of the base. The muffle is placed in the furnace, which is heated to 850°C. The rate of temperature rise is 3°C to 6°C per minute. After 90 minutes at 850°C, the stabilizing

elements are removed and the muffle is prepared for the pressing procedure.

The Press Furnace

Heat pressing of glass ceramic requires a special furnace for a controlled process; this unit has been based on the Programat P 90 (Fig 16-14). The following functions are still identical:

- Stand-by temperature
- Rate of heat rise
- Final temperature
- Vacuum on
- Vacuum off
- Holding temperature

In order to heat press glass ceramic, the following elements were added or altered:

- Enlargement of the heat dome
- Installation of a pneumatic pressure system
- Addition of reducing valve and manometer for optimal pressure control

Further control of the process is accomplished with an inductive displacement transducer mounted on the pneumatic plunger.

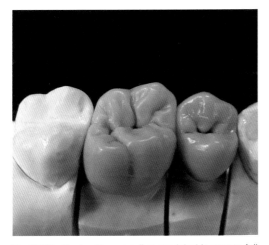

Fig 16-12 Restorations are first modeled in wax to full crown contour as for the metal casting technique. The entire procedure is performed using only one working model.

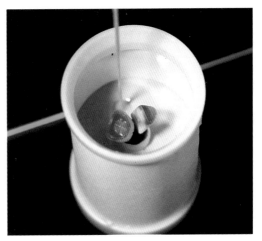

Fig 16-13 The waxed-up restorations are invested using a specially developed investment material. Its excellent expansion control allows crowns of superb precision to be fabricated.

This important sensor monitors the pressing procedure and sends an electronic signal that determines the automatic operation of the program. As soon as the pressing is finished, the voids formed by the wax burnout are filled. The plunger ceases its motion. This step is controlled by a specific microprocessor.

In order to ensure the complete formation of all distinct line angles, a certain pressure maintenance time is programmed. This problem can arise when a thin-walled mold such as a facial veneer is to be pressed.

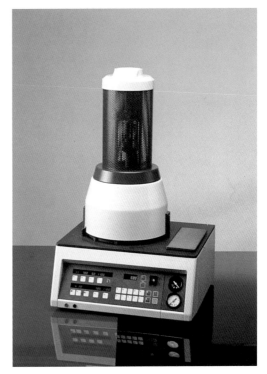

Fig 16-14 Press furnace, based on the well-tested Programat P.90.

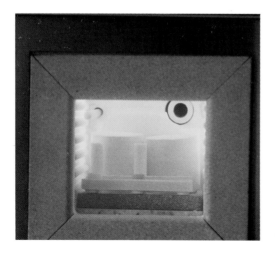

Fig 16-15 The prepared muffles are placed in a conventional preheating oven. The program corresponds to that of the metal casting technique. The rate of heat rise is 6°C per minute to 280°C, which is maintained for 60 minutes. Then the oven is heated to a final temperature of 850°C, which is held for another 60 minutes. It is recommendable that this program be run at night. The ingot and the plunger must be placed in the oven as well; it is important to have them heated at the same time as the muffles.

Pressing Technique

Preparation

The impression is cast and a master model is made just as for the metal casting technique. For the fabrication of crowns, inlays, and facial veneers, a thin coat of die spacer is applied to the gypsum cast in order to provide sufficient space for the luting agent. Furthermore, the die spacer may smooth out possible rough areas originating from the preparation.

The wax model is built up and attached to the cylindrical crucible former using 3-mm-thick wire wax. Ultimately, the special investment material is poured into the muffle. This must be done strictly according to the manufacturer's directions. Mixing of the investment with vacuum and pressure applied may prevent porosities.

Approximately 1 hour later, the crucible former is removed and the muffle is placed together with the ceramic ingots and the aluminum-oxide plunger in a preheating oven at a temperature of 850°C. The rate of temperature rise is 3°C to 6°C per minute. This temperature is maintained for a minimum of 90 minutes. A special refractory tray is sup-

plied for transfer and support of the ceramic ingots and the plunger. In general, the preheating and burn-out procedures are run at night (Fig 16-15).

Pressing Procedure

The main switch activates the press furnace. The temperature rises to the desired level (700°C). At this moment the muffle is moved from the preheating oven into the center depression of the furnace. One or two ingots are transferred from the preheating oven and placed into the muffle also. Eventually, the heat-soaked aluminum-oxide plunger is placed in the muffle and the furnace is closed (Figs 16-16 and 16-17).

The "start" button is pressed and the automatic program begins: the vacuum starts and the temperature rises at a rate of 60°C per minute; the furnace is heated until it reaches the press temperature of 1,100°C.

Once this level is achieved, it will be maintained for 20 minutes. Proper heat distribution is thereby attained, which ensures the desired temperature inside the mold. The pressing procedure starts automatically.

Usually, pressing is performed under 3.5 bar of pressure. The pressure is adjusted by

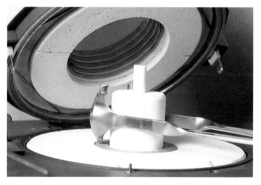 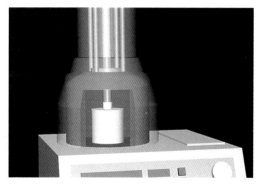

Figs 16-16 and 16-17 One to two ingots are removed from the oven and placed in the muffle. Ultimately, the aluminum oxide plunger is inserted into the muffle and the press furnace is closed.

means of a reducing valve placed at the reverse side and displayed on a manometer located on the front plate of the furnace. The distance the plunger has traveled is indicated on the display with the symbol W. As soon as the plunger travels less than 0.3 mm in 3 minutes, the program "pressure holding time" (N) is activated (Figs 16-18 to 16-22). When the sequence pressure holding time has been performed, the pressing procedure is completed. Heat and vacuum are shut off; an audible signal indicates the end of the program. The furnace is opened manually and the muffle is allowed to bench-cool to room temperature. In order to make the process adaptable to different materials, the following functions can be programmed by pressing the button P (program):

- Stand-by
  temperature   B   200°C – 850°C
- Heating rate   T   5°C – 80°C/min
- Press temperature T   200°C – 1,200°C
- Pressure
  maintenance   N   1 – 30 min
- Holding time   H   1 – 60 min
- Vacuum on   V1   0 – 1,200°C
- Vacuum off   V2   0 – 1,200°C

The programs 1 to 19 and 20 to 39 can be stored and secured by a code.

After the muffle is bench-cooled, the objects are devested. The plunger is separated with a diamond separating disk at the points of orientation that have been marked on the paper investment ring with wax prior to investing (Figs 16-23 and 16-24). After separating, the ceramic objects must be cleaned of the remaining investment. This is carefully performed using glass beads and low-pressure air abrasion (3 bar).

The IPS Die Material in Dentin Colors

A particularly favorable aspect of all-ceramic systems is translucency. It facilitates a near perfect imitation of a natural tooth by reproducing the color of the prepared die. When restoring discolored teeth or teeth with metal cores, selection of the luting agent becomes significant. A special IPS die material, which is available in nine different dentin colors, is therefore an essential component of the new technique (Figs 16-25 to 16-27).

When the preparation is finished, the color selection is made with a special shade guide.

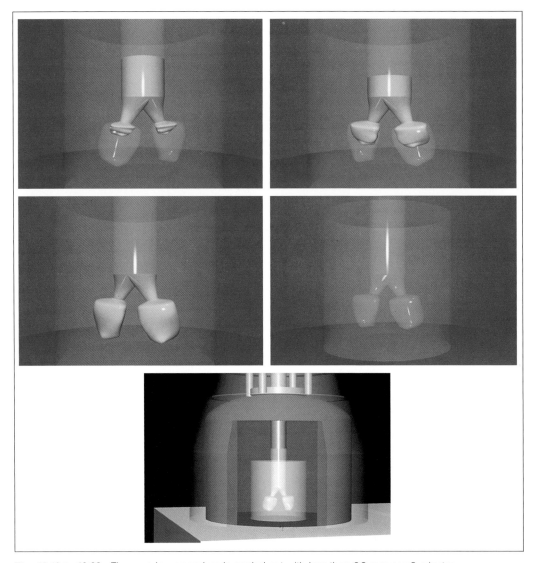

Figs 16-18 to 16-22   The pressing procedure is carried out with less than 0.3 mm per 3 minutes.

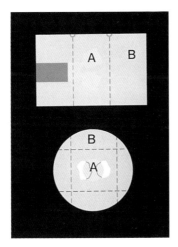
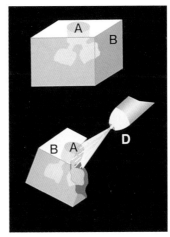

Figs 16-23 and 16-24 Devesting of the pressed ceramic objects is perhaps the most intricate step of the Empress technique. A particular method has been developed for this purpose. Prior to investing, two wax marks are placed on the paper cylinder. The first mark is made 3 to 4 mm below the wax models (A), the second mark is made above the wax-ups at the level of the plunger; the marking creates notches in the investment (C). After the pressing, the muffle (B) is cut with an oscillating saw exactly where the notches are. A disk of investment material (B), which comprises the pressed ceramic objects, is thus obtained. With four separating cuts the disk is reduced to a cube (B). Care must be exercised to work a safe distance away from the plunger (A). Gross removal of the investment is readily achieved with plastic beads and air abrasion (4 bar). When the ceramic objects are emerging from the investment, the pressure is reduced to 3 bar. The abrasive particles must be directed tangentially to the pressed restorations to prevent fracturing.

The dental technician receives the impression and the selected color of the prepared tooth. Using a light-cured die material, an appropriate IPS resin die can be formed.

By means of staining as well as layering, the color of the natural teeth can be mimicked. The die can also serve as an aid to handling the crown while coloring or building up the contour. The die is removed prior to each firing and repositioned after cooling off.

Shade Selection of the Ceramic Ingot for the Layering Technique

The scheme we adhere to when working with metal ceramic is to begin with a saturated color in the center and advance to the periphery with less saturated ones (see chapter 10, "Processing and Natural Layering of Metal Ceramic"). This technique creates a sense of depth despite thin porcelain layers and metal framework.

Empress ceramic offers a simpler solution, because there is no metal or aluminum substructure; thus there is more reflection from the core. It is therefore not necessary to apply several layers of dentin porcelain to achieve this sense of depth. The dentin core itself suffices to create the desired effect, because the light can penetrate without being reflected by the natural tooth.

The color selected for the ceramic ingot must be as close as possible to the natural tooth, however a slightly more saturated hue may be chosen. The more important the build-up of the incisal region, the less saturated the selected color should be. It should be kept in mind that it may seem relatively simple to select hue and saturation, but it is much more difficult to determine color brilliance.

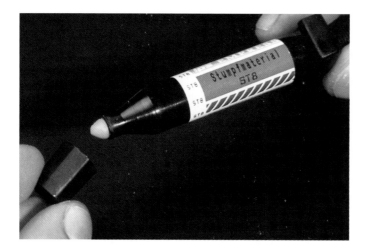

Fig 16-25 For the build-up of the special resin die, light-curing resin is used.

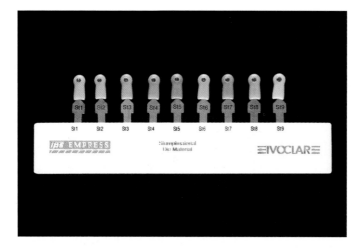

Fig 16-26 The die material is available in nine different colors. The dentist selects the color of the die according to this shade guide.

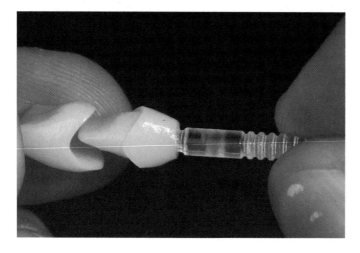

Fig 16-27 The pressed porcelain crown serves as an aid for duplicating the original prepared tooth in light-curing resin. The ceramist is thus able to evaluate the color of the prepared tooth and take the result into consideration during the build-up. In addition, the resin die serves as a handle, making staining and layering procedures easier.

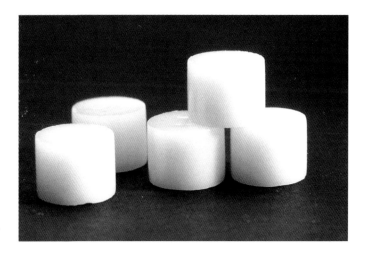

Fig 16-28 Ingots of varying transparencies used for modeling.

For this reason, when working with the Empress system, it is important not to select a color that is too gray, because it will later be impossible to correct the brilliance. In most cases, the pressed core represents two thirds of the entire restoration.

Staining Technique

In order to supply color to the crown of a molar, inlay, or facial veneer, the surface can be stained. For this purpose, ceramic ingots of different transparencies can be used (Fig 16-28). Transparency is more significant with inlays or facial veneers than with crowns; the latter rely more on opacity.

The surface stains are supplied according to the colors of teeth; this makes reproduction of natural colors considerably easier (Fig 16-29). A range of 15 surface stains can reproduce all colors of teeth. Moreover, there are eight "intense" staining pastes for characterization. In order to stain the ceramic objects in the desired manner, three to five coats of surface stain must be applied and successively vacuum-fired for 2 minutes at 850°C. A glaze bake completes the firing cycle. The different steps of fabrication of a premolar crown are depicted in Fig 16-30.

As described previously, the first step is the fabrication of a special working die that has the same color as the one selected by the dentist. The crown is seated on this die and colored. It is important to remove the special resin die before the firing. After cooling off, the crown is reseated, the color match is checked, and the staining process is continued. The die should be coated with a drop of glycerine to prevent the incorporation of air at the fitting surface, as this would cause refraction and hence change the color.

The technique of staining the surface (ie, a mere superficial coloring) is less esthetic and less innovative, although it can prove quite helpful with posterior teeth where accurate contour and occlusal relations are important. Furthermore, this technique is much easier for student ceramists to use.

Layering Technique

The layering technique is interesting and innovative because the color emerges from deep inside, based on the dentin core. Ceramic ingots are precolored according to the shade guide by Ivoclar or Vita (Fig 16-31). This system does not limit the ceramist's creativity. In order to imitate the vital ap-

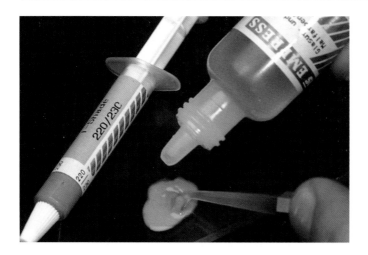

Fig 16-29 Stains are marketed in a ready-to-use creamy consistency. The tubes clearly show their colors, which corresponds to the shade guides of Vita and Ivoclar.

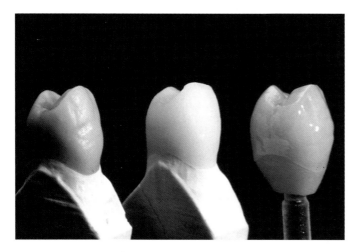

Fig 16-30 Prior to the application of the stain, the restoration is built up to full contour *(left)*. The crown is first pressed with transparent ingots *(middle)* and then stained *(right)*.

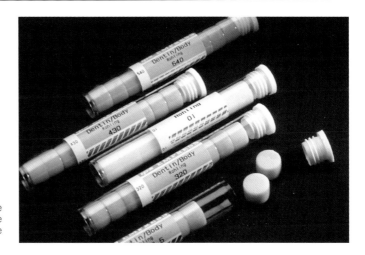

Fig 16-31 The layering technique requires ceramic ingots that are precolored according to the shade guides of Vita and Ivoclar.

pearance of natural teeth, this technique can be used for very simple tasks as well as for complex build-ups.

A prerequisite for sufficient resistance to fracture is the harmonious adjustment between the layered ceramic and the pressed ceramic. The coefficient of thermal expansion of the layered ceramic is inferior to that of the pressed ceramic. Therefore, during the cooling off after the firing, compressive stress develops at the interface of the pressed ceramic, which compensates the tensile stress under application of load (Figs 16-32 and 16-33).

Fabrication of the dentin core. An essential property of this material is that the core provides the basic color, because there is no metal or aluminum substructure. It is essential to use a variety of incisal porcelains and stains to mimic natural teeth.

There is one condition that should not be overlooked: full contour must already be established in wax. The contour of the cervical third or the proximal portion, for instance (the latter is particularly significant because it determines the interproximal space), is not altered during the ensuing firings. Knowing the difficulties that exist in forming these parts of metal ceramic restorations, especially for anterior teeth, the eminent advantage of the discussed technique

is clear: all these details are predetermined (Fig 16-34).

The dentin core can be premodeled in wax. When the ceramist specifies the color, he knows exactly where to leave some space for effects. He can fabricate a dentin core that represents only one third of shape and function of the tooth to be restored. He can also adapt the dentin core to the shape of the tooth and the age of the patient, which will mostly be the case for anterior teeth. The easy (and reasonable) way is to establish these details in wax rather than to shape the pressed material later by grinding or milling (Figs 16-35 and 16-36). The prepared dies are coated with beige-colored die spacer to prevent the color of the semitranslucent core from exerting too much influence. One or two coats of die spacer can be applied depending on the dentist's preference and the type of preparation (Fig 16-37).

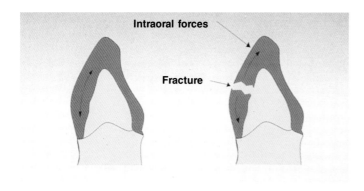

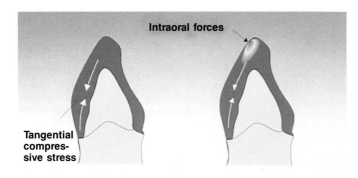

Figs 16-32 and 16-33 *(above)* Added tensile stress causes fracture. Functional (occlusal) loads can cause crowns without compressive prestress or that are not subjected to tensile stress to fracture. *(below)* Compressive stress reduces tensile stress. Crowns with compressive prestress are more resistant to functional (occlusal) loading. According to Anusavice.

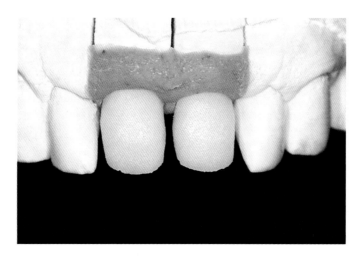

Fig 16-34 One advantage of the layering technique is the ability to form the proximal contour and the embrasure at the dentin core stage.

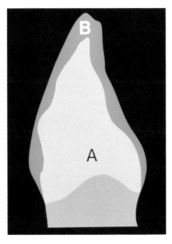

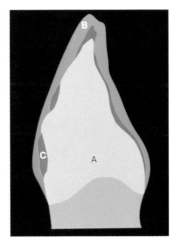

Fig 16-35 Study of the shape of a dentin core *(A)*. Any tooth, and subsequently every restoration, is an individual case for which the cross section should be individually adapted. *(B)* The incisal edge with regard to the layering technique. There is no strict rule. Regardless of whether the layer is thin or thick, if the ceramist has to apply only a thin layer, his work will be done quicker and easier, provided the basic color has already been determined by the dentin core.

Fig 16-36 The material marked *(C)* has been applied for the wash and effect bake. The small amounts ensure that this can be rapidly performed. These layers are applied beneath the incisal layer *(B)*.

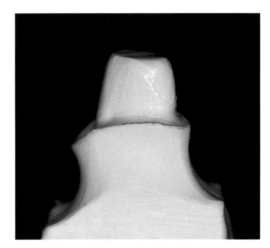

Fig 16-37 A coat of beige-colored die spacer has been applied to the die in order to protect the porcelain crown from too much undesirable color influence when seated. (Die spacer varnish by Symphyse, Marseilles, France.)

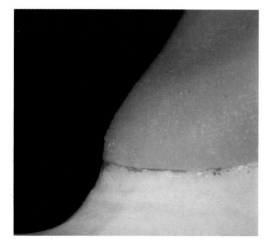

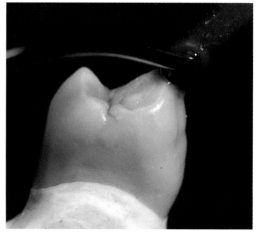

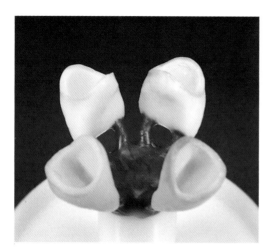

Fig 16-38 The quality of the investment as well as our ability to manipulate expansion facilitate restorations of perfect fit.

Fig 16-39 The pressing procedure requires one piece of 3-mm wax wire.

Fig 16-40 Four restorations (of identical color) can be placed in the muffle at a time.

The wax-up of the dentin core slightly resembles that of a metal substructure. On the one hand, we can work on a traditionally prepared primary model; on the other hand, we can refer to a wax-up that is as precise as possible.

The accuracy of the pressed core depends on skillful manipulation of the wax as well as exact dosage of the investment. Because of our ability to manipulate expansion, it is possible to achieve a high degree of accuracy (Fig 16-38).

After the wax model has been completed and the cervical margin inspected with a magnifying glass, a 3-mm-thick wax wire is attached to the free end of the model perpendicular to the tooth axis (Fig 16-39).

The wax models are placed on the base. Not more than four pieces should be pressed simultaneously; furthermore, they must be of identical color. The length of the sprue should not exceed 3 mm (Fig 16-40). The muffle is made of paper with the upper end strengthened by a removable plastic ring.

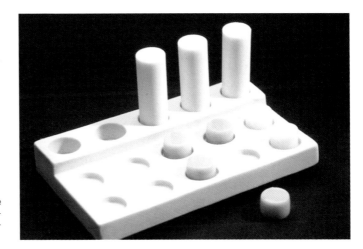

Fig 16-41 Each pressing procedure requires preheating of an aluminum-oxide plunger and the corresponding ingots, together with the muffle.

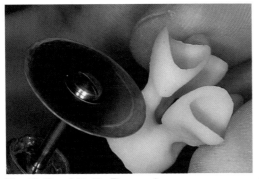 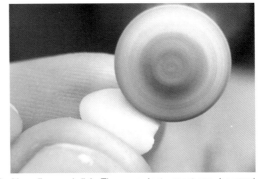

Figs 16-42 and 16-43 The pressing sprues are removed with a diamond disk. The same instrument may be used to refine details on the incisal edges without breaking the porcelain. The attachment points are smoothed with an abrasive stone (see chapter 19).

Inside the muffle, points of orientation are marked with wax: one above the wax models, the other below the level of the sprue former. These marks, which are in a negative position to the muffle, prove useful in estimating the position of the pressed ceramic objects. When the bulk of the investment is later removed with a saw, the restoration will thus be protected. The investing is done traditionally: the muffle is placed into a pressure curing vessel for 20 minutes, thus preventing the incorporation of air.

Programming of the preheating oven is similar to that used for the metal casting technique and the usual casting ring. The muffles are placed, together with the casting rings for metal casting, in the preheating oven overnight.

The precolored ceramic ingots and the aluminum oxide plunger are placed together in the preheating oven (Fig 16-41). The pressing procedure is simple. The press furnace is heated to 700°C. The muffle is moved from the preheating oven into the center of the

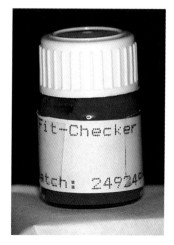

Fig 16-44 To fully seat the pressed crowns on the dies, a special friction paste is used. The die is coated with a thin film of the paste. Multiple repositioning of the restoration creates undesirable interferences that must be eliminated.

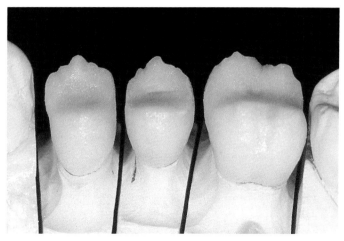

Fig 16-45 The first porcelain layer can be applied. Attention must be paid to the shape of the dentin core. It requires only a relatively thin layer to establish full crown contour.

furnace. One or two ceramic ingots are placed into the muffle. Eventually, the pre-heated plunger is inserted into the muffle. The programmed operation takes approximately 35 minutes. After cooling off, only the investment needs to be removed.

It is strongly recommended that a hammer not be used for devesting. Instead, a saw should be used to recover the pressed bulk with the crowns from the investment; only a small amount of investment should remain around the crowns. Air abrasion with a pressure of 4 bar and plastic beads will clean the restoration thoroughly; the interior surface is treated only with a pressure of 3 bar.

The sprues are separated with a diamond disk. The remaining excess at the attachment points is removed with an abrasive stone (Figs 16-42 and 16-43). The porcelain cores are then cleaned. If friction is too tight or slight undercuts appear, the surfaces must be adjusted by grinding. Again, magnifying glasses and friction paste are used for this inspection (Fig 16-44).

Layering. After the porcelain cores have been reseated on the dies, they are treated with low-pressure air abrasion using aluminum oxide and are steamed for degreasing. The cleaned ceramic cores are ready for the porcelain layering (Fig 16-45).

- First bake (wash and effect bake). The first step is a wash and effect firing sequence. It should create a strong bond between the two different materials, which possess compatible coefficients of thermal expansion.

A neutral ceramic powder is mixed with a metal oxide liquid. The mix is applied in a thin coat to the entire surface of the porcelain core. At the same time, attention must be paid to the dentin effects and the free margins (Figs 16-46 and 16-47). In the case of insufficient space, it is possible to create certain effects by surface staining. This method is recommended for facial veneers.

The firing is performed in a ceramic furnace, and the program is similar to that of a bisque bake for metal ceramic. A slow cooling is the

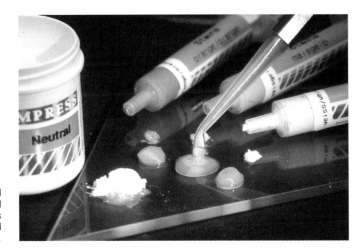

Fig 16-46   The powders are mixed with glazing liquid for the wash and effect bake. This measure increases the refractive index of light and renders the colors more conspicuous.

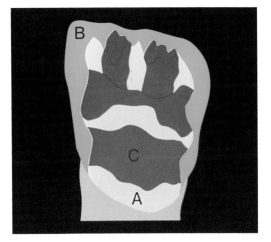

Fig 16-47   A dentin core cross section. The dentin core (A) is already covered by successive layers for the wash and effect bake (C). The incisal edge (B) should have been built up according to the layering technique.

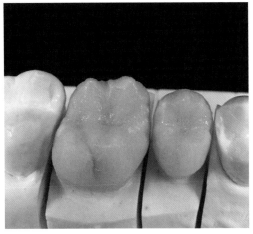

Fig 16-48   Restorations after the wash and effect bake. Attention should be paid to the subtle shade effects that have been incorporated beneath the enamel layer.

only measure that must be ensured. Not before the temperature is reduced to 300°C can the crown be removed from the furnace (Fig 16-48).

- Second bake. Prior to completion of the build-up, the crown must be degreased once more by steam cleaning. The last step of the modeling is performed quickly because the amount that needs to be

applied has only the thickness of the enamel layer of a natural tooth.

This can be done following the principle of lateral segmentation (Fig 16-49). The ceramic should not be overcontoured, because the thin porcelain layer will only be subject to light refraction. The programming of the furnace is identical to the wash and effect bake.

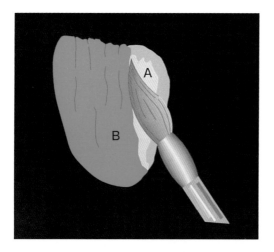

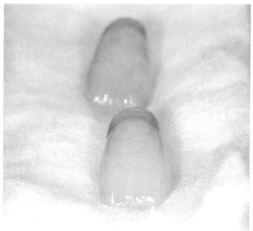

Fig 16-49   The incisal third *(B)* is modeled according to the lateral segmentation technique if the Empress system is used. *(A)* The dentin core.

Fig 16-50   For the glaze bake the restorations are placed on a nonflammable cotton-wool pad.

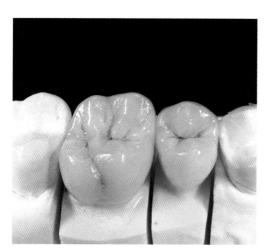

Fig 16-51   Empress crowns after polishing.

In general, one glaze bake is sufficient after the bisque bake. The contour that is obtained after the second bake represents the final contour of the restoration.

- Third bake (minimum glaze bake). The restoration is only slightly colored because the effects have already been established at earlier stages. Surface staining can only create superficial effects, similar to those on natural teeth (eg, discoloration at the floor of fissures, discoloration at proximal surfaces and at the cervical area). For the glaze bake, the restoration is placed on a nonflammable cotton-wool pad (Fig 16-50) and air-fired at a temperature slightly lower than that in the preceding programs. Ultimately, the restoration is polished (Fig 16-51; see chapter 19).

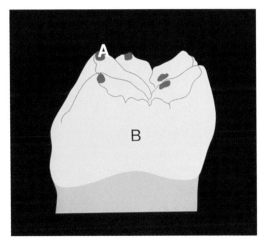 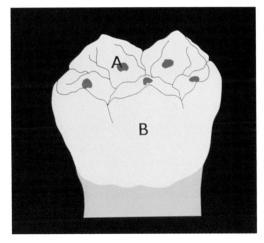

Figs 16-52 and 16-53 Functional relations and occlusal contacts can be established in wax when posterior teeth are to be restored.

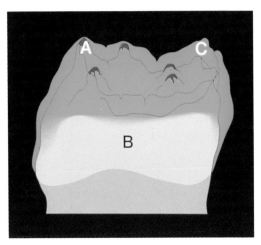 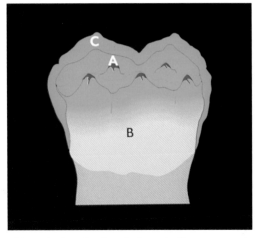

Figs 16-54 and 16-55 After thorough studies of function, all important occlusal contacts or dentin cones can be preserved. The wax model can be sufficiently reduced so that enough space will be provided for the layering technique. The pressed dentin core exhibits an established dimensional stability while the occlusal relations and contacts are fully preserved.

The Dentin Core for Restorations of Posterior Teeth

Functional and occlusal aspects must be assessed carefully when posterior teeth are to be restored. It is important to study function in order to accurately restore morphology and occlusal relations.

When using the layering technique, the restoration will inevitably be reduced, thus sufficient space will be created for the enamel porcelain. It may appear that our striving for occlusal reproduction has been in vain, because we have to reduce now, but this is not so! All occlusal contacts should be preserved and only as much wax as absolutely necessary should be removed from around these points. They are preserved in

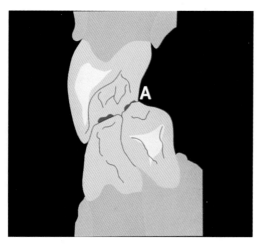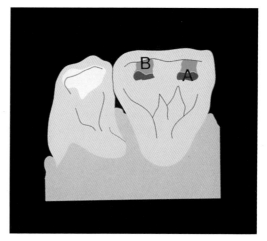

Figs 16-56 and 16-57 With restorations of anterior teeth, the occlusal contacts *(A)* and the incisal guidance *(B)* can both be built up in wax. They will be preserved through the firing cycle of the layered ceramic build-up.

their original contour, but after the reduction they look similar to dentin cones.

During fabrication of the restoration, the enamel is applied incrementally without covering the occlusal contacts. There will be no firing shrinkage, and the occlusion, adjusted beforehand, is preserved accurately. The dentin color is covered by the surrounding incisal porcelain and thus "camouflaged." This approach is thus interesting for the ceramist who has experienced difficulties in achieving accurate occlusal relations despite the bake and subsequent shrinkage (Figs 16-52 to 16-55).

The Dentin Core for Anterior Restorations

It is also advisable to establish a wax-up in complete contour for maxillary anterior restorations. The incisal guidance can be readily studied in the articulator (Figs 16-56 and 16-57). In order to facilitate the layering technique, the restoration is reduced while the occlusal contacts and the guiding paths are preserved (Figs 16-58 and 16-59). After the dentin-colored restorations are pressed, a try-in can be performed to inspect the inter-

proximal spaces, occlusal relations, and incisal guidance. The dentist can adjust the incisal guidance perfectly by grinding in the mouth. The occlusal contacts and the incisal guidance are preserved in their exact form; no deformation occurs through firing, which saves much work. These fixed markings are of great help for the ceramist and become inconspicuous after the application of the incisal porcelain once the crowns are completed.

For esthetic reasons it is possible to perform a trial seating prior to the firing. For this purpose the full contour of the enamel is established in colored wax (Figs 16-60 and 16-61). The dentist then inspects the marginal fit, functional aspects (thanks to the markings), shape, and color. This technique offers a variety of solutions for the ambitious technician who strives for excellent results.

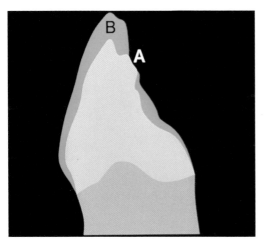

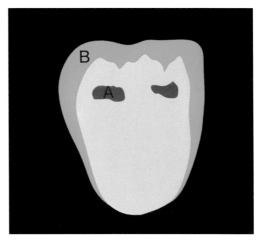

Fig 16-58 Sagittal cross section of a pressed ceramic core. The lingual contact was intentionally preserved. Thus, we can also preserve the occlusal relations that have been established during the wax-up in the articulator. *(A)* Occlusal contact of the pressed core. *(B)* The contour that remains to be built up with the layering technique. If the contour has been reduced in the same manner as shown, the layer can be rapidly rebuilt.

Fig 16-59 Lingual view of the pressed core. The incisal region was completely waxed-up prior to the pressing. *(A)* Lingual occlusal contact. *(B)* Region restored by means of the layering technique. The dentin core is stable. After the layering bake, shrinkage may occur: the material within the build-up can be controlled before the firing.

Figs 16-60 and 16-61 For inspection purposes of marginal adaptation, function, and esthetics, the pressed dentin cores can be trial seated in the patient's mouth, using colored wax, after the wax-up of the enamel layer.

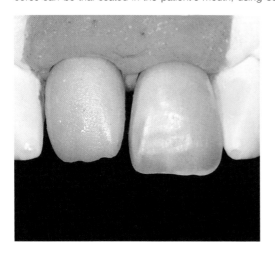

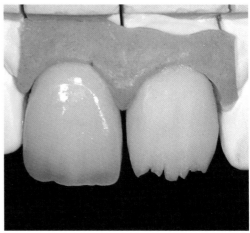

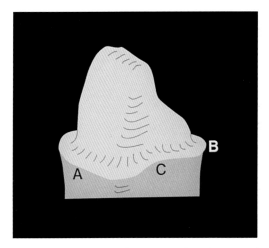

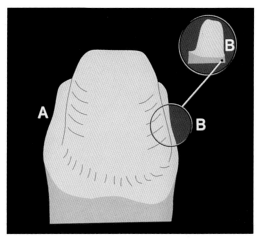

Fig 16-62 The preparation for a tooth to be restored with an Empress crown resembles that of a porcelain "jacket" crown. The shoulder must be rounded at the transition from the floor of the shoulder to the vertical portion of the tooth. The finish line (A-B-C), on the other hand, must be a clean, right-angled edge to provide for a perfect marginal fit of the crown.

Fig 16-63 The shoulder must not be absolutely regular but circumferential. Areas that lack clear shoulder definition must be corrected to prevent fracture of the pressed crown (B). Furthermore, too much variation in width of the shoulder (A and B) is undesirable for a material subjected to multiple firings.

Fig 16-64 Occlusal view of a tooth preparation for an Empress crown. The width may vary but it must be circumferential. (A) The labial portion should be 1 to 1.5 mm wide. (C and D) With regard to the proximal portion it is difficult to provide for more than absolutely necessary, because the pulp is in close proximity (0.6 mm). (B) The lingual portion should be 1 mm wide.

Fig 16-65 The angle of a full shoulder can vary from 90° to 135° at the finish line. Because of great stability of the reinforced porcelain, prominent angles must be avoided (B, C, D). The surface of the prepared tooth should be smoothed in all areas except for the well-defined edge of the finish line (A).

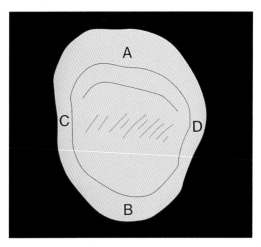

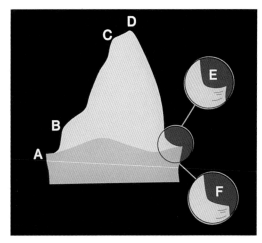

Tooth Preparation
for Pressed Ceramic Restorations
(Figs 16-62 to 16-70)

For pressed ceramic restorations, either a 90°
shoulder preparation with rounded line angles
or a 135° chamfer preparation is imperative.
The preparation should have rounded edges.
A thickness of 1.5 mm to 2 mm (occlusal or
incisal) must be ensured. The width of the
shoulder should be 1 to 1.5 mm (labial and
proximal) and at least 1 mm (lingual). Thickness of the remaining dentin should not be
less than 0.6 mm. The preparation margin
must be right-angled to ensure a perfect
marginal fit. On the lingual surface, minimum
thickness is 1 mm. Less than that would increase the crown's fracture potential, particularly in occlusal regions.

Figures 16-71 to 16-89 show clinical results
using the pressed ceramic technique.

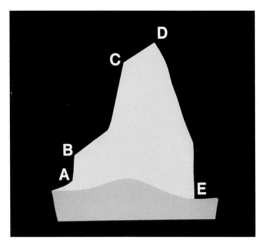

Fig 16-66   This is an example of how the preparation
for a pressed crown should *not* be performed.

Figs 16-67 and 16-68   Adequate preparations that are suitable for pressed ceramic. Rounded preparation (C);
rounded shoulder (A); clean, right-angled finish line (B).

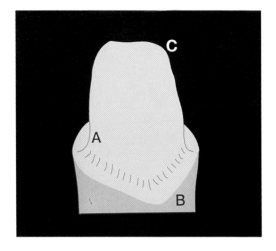

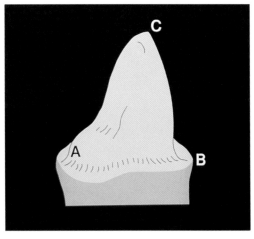

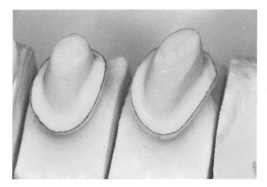

Fig 16-69 Excellent preparations for pressed ceramic crowns. Preparation of vital teeth for a 48-year-old patient. (Preparations courtesy of Dr Thierry Jeannin, Orange, France.)

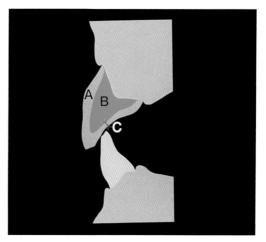

Fig 16-70 Minimum thickness of the lingual portion for an Empress restoration is 1 mm *(C)*. Insufficient reduction of tooth structure, particularly regarding occlusal contacts, may result in fracturing of the restoration.

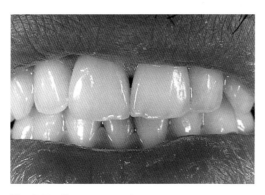

Fig 16-71 Empress ceramic crown on tooth 11. This is the very first restoration fabricated in our laboratory using the new technique. (Courtesy of Dr Michel Canazzi, Caderousse, France.)

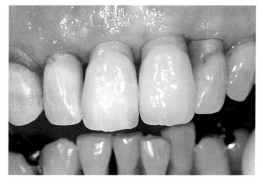

Fig 16-72 Empress ceramic crowns on teeth 11 and 21. (Courtesy of Dr Michel Canazzi, Caderousse, France.)

Figs 16-73 and 16-74 Optec ceramic crowns on teeth 11, 12, 21, and 22. (Courtesy of Dr Novak, Avignon, France.)

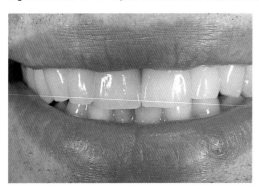

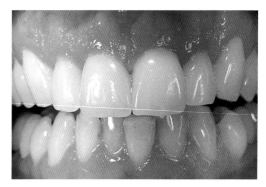

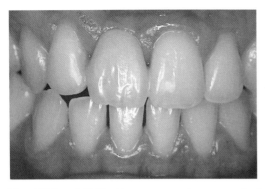
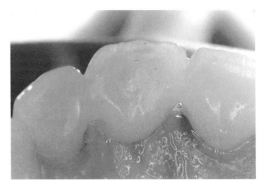

Figs 16-75 and 16-76 Empress ceramic crown on tooth 11 and two lingual veneers on teeth 21 and 12. (Courtesy of Dr Luc Portalier, Aix-en-Provence, France.)

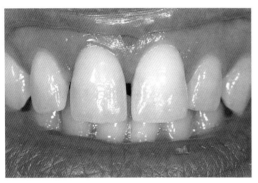

Fig 16-77 Empress ceramic crown on tooth 11. (Courtesy of Dr Yeche, Avignon, France.)

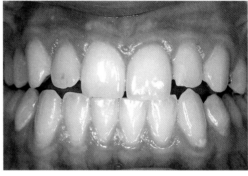

Fig 16-78 Empress ceramic crown on tooth 21. The surface structure is not correctly reproduced; light reflection differs in comparison to the adjacent tooth. (Courtesy of Dr Daniel Gleyzolle, Avignon, France.)

Fig 16-79 Four Empress ceramic crowns on teeth 11, 12, 21, and 22. The teeth are restored with a ceramic post and core. Even though only one porcelain powder was used for the layering of these crowns, the result is satisfying. (Courtesy of Dr Daniel Gleyzolle, Avignon, France.)

Fig 16-80 Empress ceramic crowns on tooth 12. (Courtesy of Dr Thierry Jeannin, Orange, France.)

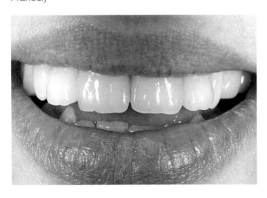
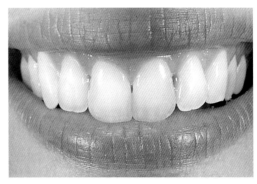

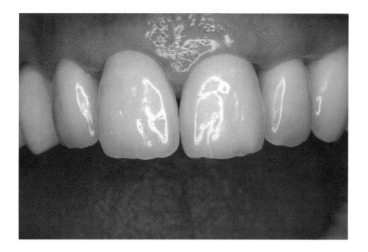

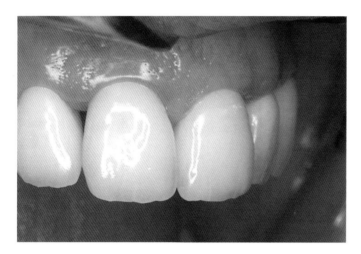

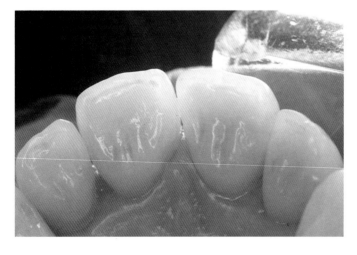

Figs 16-81 to 16-83 Empress ceramic crowns on teeth 11, 12, 13, 21, and 22. (Courtesy of Dr Thierry Jeannin, Orange, France.).

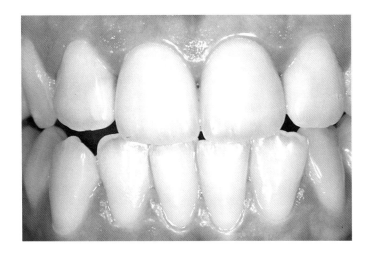

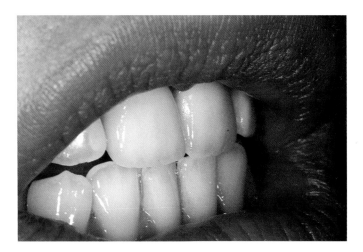

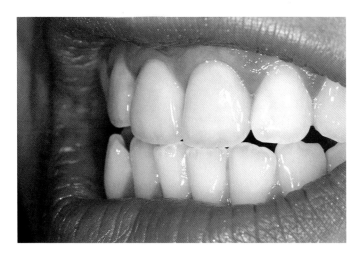

Figs 16-84 to 16-86 Empress ceramic crowns on teeth 11 and 21. (Courtesy of Dr Michel Canazzi, Caderousse, France.)

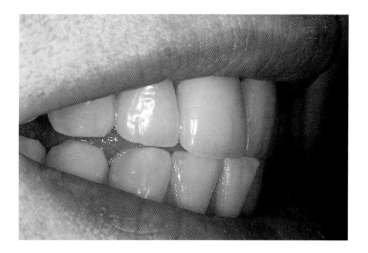

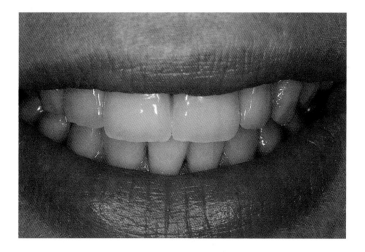

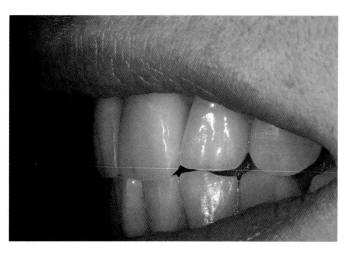

Figs 16-87 to 16-89 Empress ceramic crowns on teeth 12, 11, and 22. (Courtesy of Dr Michel Canazzi, Caderousse, France.)

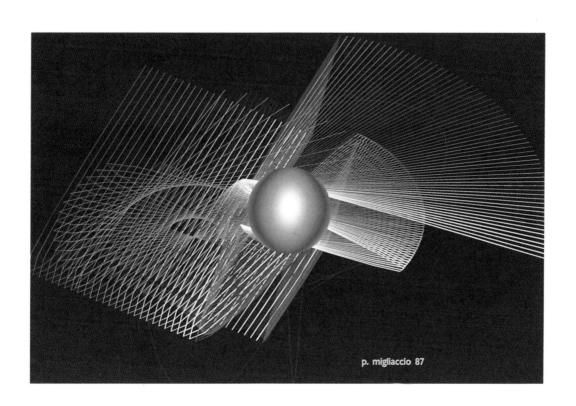

17 Post and Core in Ceramics

Empress porcelain in general offers maximum esthetic potential for the restoration of vital teeth. At times, however, it may be necessary to first restore a tooth with a post and core. A metal post and core impairs the esthetic properties of porcelain materials because of the reflection of light by the metal. For that reason, we fabricate a post and core using dentin porcelain that is supported by a mini-substructure consisting of metal.

When we first experimented, we simply coated the metal with opaque porcelain. This prevented gray reflections but still the light was "retarded." Clinical results were satisfactory and very similar to metal ceramic restorations with all their disadvantages; the major problem was metamerism.

Today we fabricate post and core restorations differently. First we fabricate a metal mini-substructure to support the porcelain. The casting of these substructures is identical to that for metal ceramic frameworks. We build up the contour of the core using a saturated dentin porcelain. This should mimic the color of the prepared tooth or that of the pulp. These small substructures are quickly fabricated, and so is the modeling. The fabrication is performed as follows.

① **Fabrication of metal substructures for ceramic post and core for maxillary canines and central incisors.** The post as well as the base of the core, both supporting the two vertical cones, are made of metal. The cones are fabricated with standardized 0.1-mm-thick wire. The richmond plateau should be as thin as possible. It is always slightly retracted from the finish line, thus providing space for a circumferential shoulder. The two cones are positioned mesially and distally with sufficient distance in between. Light can thus circulate through the core (Fig 17-1).

② **Fabrication of metal substructures for ceramic post and core for lateral incisors.** For small and narrow teeth it is not possible to position two cones mesially and distally. Consequently, only one cone is planned to suit the substructure. Here again the richmond plateau should be as thin as possible in order to provide space for the circumferential shoulder (Fig 17-2).

③ **Fabrication of metal substructures for a ceramic post and core for premolars.** Substructures for premolars are fabricated in a manner nearly identical to that for maxillary canines and central incisors. The difference is that the two cones are positioned in a faciolingual direction. Again enough space must be left for the circumferential shoulder (Fig 17-3).

④ **Fabrication of metal substructures for a ceramic post and core for molars.** A post and core for molars frequently requires the positioning of an additional retaining element, which may prove difficult. The posts and the richmond plateau are fabricated in the aforementioned manner. The retaining element must be removable and made of metal to support the porcelain. Two cones are positioned in the facial portion, leaving sufficient space for the circumferential shoulder (Fig 17-4).

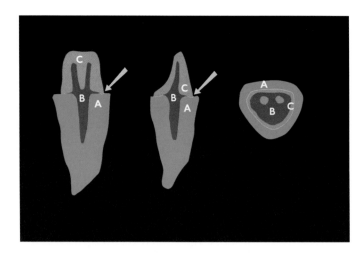

Figs 17-1 to 17-4 Ceramic post and core fabrication for porcelain jacket crowns.

Figs 17-1 Ceramic post and core for a maxillary central incisor. *(A)* Root; *(B)* metal substructure with two reinforcing cones placed mesially and distally; *(C)* porcelain (dentin material). The periphery of the substructure should be porcelain to avoid gray reflections.

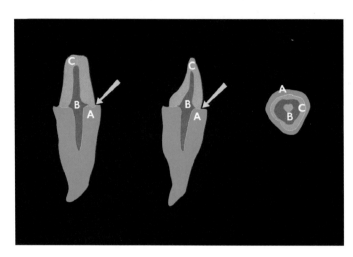

Fig 17-2 Ceramic post and core for maxillary lateral incisors and for mandibular incisors. Fabrication is identical to that described in Fig 17-1, except for the fact that only one reinforcing cone is used.

Fabrication of a Porcelain Post and Core

The ceramic substructure is not built up with just any porcelain. First we must select the color of the porcelain in the patient's mouth. If the tooth is destroyed as far as the gingival crest, an orange porcelain is chosen in order to mimic the pulp deep inside. The ceramic layering for a post and core is performed in the same manner as for metal ceramic restorations. The metal is treated, opaque is applied for masking, and successively all other layers of porcelain are applied. For reasons of better integration, the margin of the post and core is built up in porcelain (approximately 0.3 mm). This masks the gray reflections stemming from the richmond plateau (see Figs 17-1 to 17-4).

If the Empress system is used, such ceramic post and core restorations are a good option. Esthetic qualities are preserved by the almost unimpeded circulation of light. The metal cones reduce light penetration by only 10% to 15% (Fig 17-5). However, these metal cones supply the much-needed mechanical strength to the post and core.

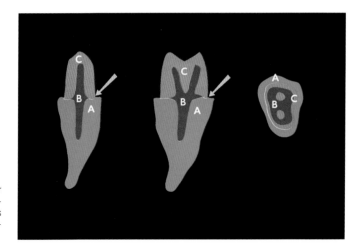

Fig 17-3 Ceramic post and core for premolars. *(A)* Root; *(B)* metal substructure with reinforcing cones placed facially and lingually; *(C)* porcelain (dentin material).

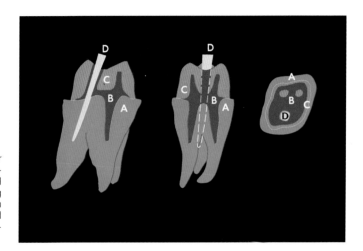

Fig 17-4 Ceramic post and core for molars showing an additional retaining element. *(A)* Root; *(B)* metal substructure with two reinforcing cones placed facially; *(C)* porcelain (dentin material); *(D)* additional (metal) post that is separately attached to the root and the core.

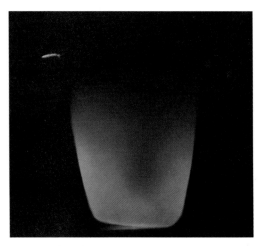

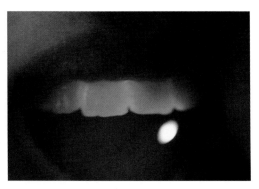

Fig 17-6 Four Empress ceramic crowns on four ceramic post and core structures. Light penetrability is satisfactory.

Fig 17-5 Ceramic post and core for maxillary lateral incisor in situ. The metal cones decrease light penetrability only by 10% to 15%.

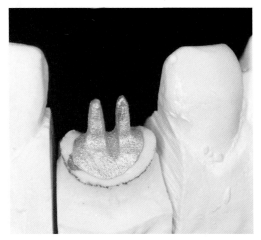

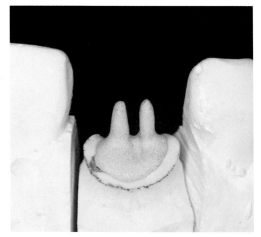

Fig 17-7 Fabrication of a ceramic post and core structure for tooth 11. The metal substructure has two reinforcing cones and one coat of covering gold.

Fig 17-8 Opaque applied to the substructure.

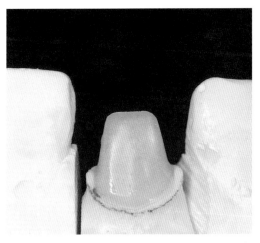

Fig 17-9 Two firings are necessary to give the dentin porcelain core the correct shape.

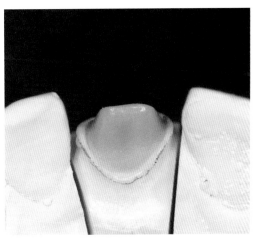

Fig 17-10 Lingual view of the ceramic post and core. Note the circumferential shoulder for the all-ceramic crown.

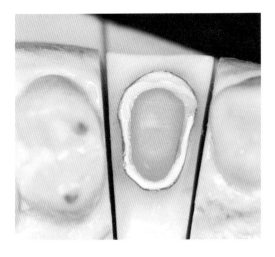

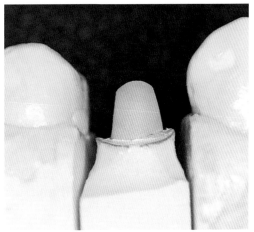

Fig 17-11 Occlusal view of a ceramic post and core for tooth 24 with a facial and a lingual metal cone.

Fig 17-12 Buccal view of the ceramic post and core. The yellow-orange color should simulate the color of the pulp, which acts iridescent inside the restoration. This effect is quite similar to that found in natural teeth.

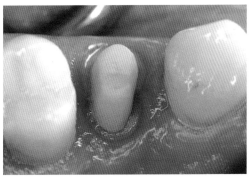

Fig 17-13 Ceramic post and core in situ. (Courtesy of Dr Luc Portalier, Aix-en-Provence, France.)

18   Facial Veneers

With modern dental techniques we are able to offer a variety of restorative solutions to our patients. The fabrication of porcelain veneers is certainly one of the most pioneering methods. To change a smile, to mask conspicuous discolorations, to correct malaligned teeth with just a few millimeters of porcelain is a difficult and challenging task for the dentist as well as for the dental technician. How satisfying, on the other hand, when the work is successfully completed! The fabrication of esthetic veneers requires profound knowledge about the use and color of porcelain, and it is certainly one of the most intricate of restorations.

Our first facial veneers were produced on refractory dies according to the method for inlay fabrication. Instantly, we could boast very satisfying results. The porcelain used was traditional (IPS Ivoclar) (Figs 18-1 to 18-8). The great disadvantages, however, were the extended periods of preheating and cooling. In addition, it was impossible to perform a correction bake after the investment had been removed. A genuine problem is that during fabrication there is no control of the opacity of the porcelain, especially if strong discolorations are to be masked. Investment material, which is white or gray, will not be a proper guideline as to what color would be underlying a restoration.

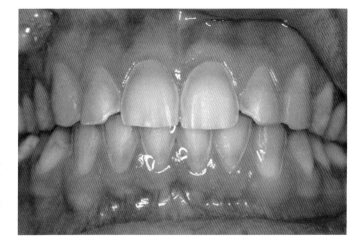

Fig 18-1   Preparation for 20 veneers (note the delicate preparation). If discolorations are to be masked, a thickness of only a few tenths of a millimeter is supplied for the layer. Ceramic: Classic IPS and Maverick, Ivoclar. (Preparations courtesy of Dr Luc Portalier, Aix-en-Provence, France.)

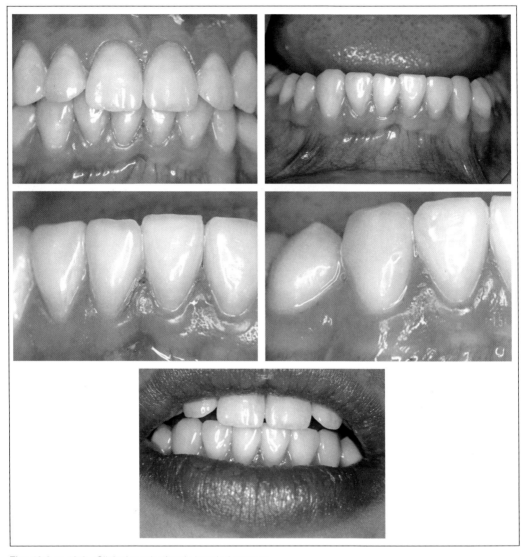

Figs 18-2 to 18-6 Clinical result of resin-bonded veneers.

As soon as these restorations are recovered from the investment, their brittleness requires extremely careful handling in order to prevent fracturing. Another problem is the establishment of correct proximal contacts, because it is usually impossible to separate the single die on the special refractory model.

These combined problems naturally influenced our decision to use the Empress ceramic system for facial veneers, too. It offers better manipulation and makes color control considerably easier. Currently, we use only the layering technique with the Empress system. This requires preparations according to the principle of conservation of tooth structure; the incisal reduction for anterior teeth is 1 mm. The most common preparation techniques are shown in Figs 18-9 to 18-12.

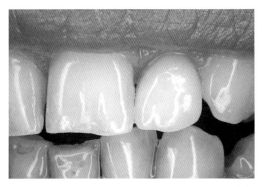
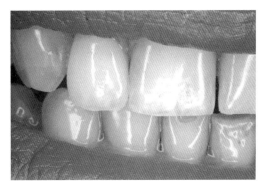

Figs 18-7 and 18-8 Two ceramic veneers on teeth 22 and 12. Ceramic: Classic IPS and Maverick, Ivoclar.

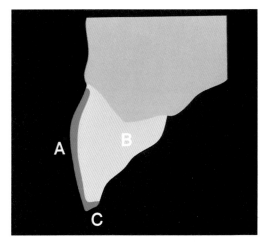

Fig 18-9 Sagittal cross section of a tooth *(B)* and a veneer *(A)*. Note the space created at the incisal edge for the layering.

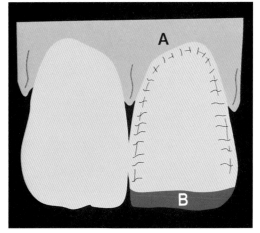

Fig 18-10 Labial view of a preparation for a ceramic veneer. The preparation is performed according to the principle of conservation of tooth structure; the reduction is ultra-thin. The finish line presents a groove. *(B)* The area of incisal reduction (approximately 1 to 1.5 mm).

Figs 18-11 and 18-12 Preparation for a veneer. (Courtesy of Dr Luc Portalier, Aix-en-Provence, France.)

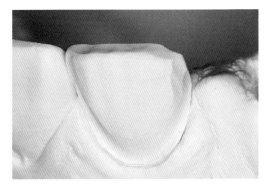
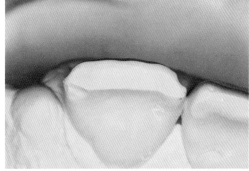

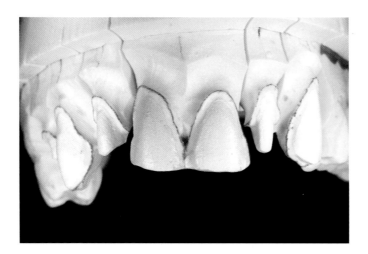

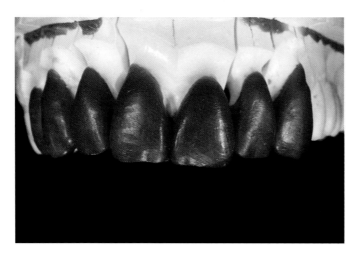

Figs 18-13 and 18-14 Preparations for Empress veneers and Empress crowns. The esthetics can be evaluated at the wax model stage.

The Empress Method for Porcelain Facial Veneers

Fabrication of the wax models. After two coats of beige-colored die spacer have been applied to the dies, wax veneers are fabricated on the working cast. It is usually impossible to separate the dies, because the proximal contacts have not been included in the preparation. During the establishment of the contour, an esthetic wax-up method is used (Figs 18-13 and 18-14). The special burn-out wax is eliminated to 100%. During the preheating of the mold, the wax must be totally eliminated, so that no residue can be incorporated into the later pressed ceramic. While the wax-up is performed, we can study the functional relations in the articulator; at this stage the correct incisal guidance is established. If the veneers are too thin, we slightly overcontour the wax-up prior to investing. A thickness of 1 mm is sufficient for the pressing procedure. A 3-mm sprue is attached to the incisal edge (Fig 18-15). Four veneers can be placed in one Empress muffle

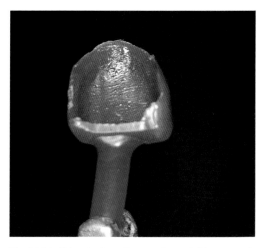

Fig 18-15 Prior to investing, a 3-mm-thick sprue is attached to the incisal edge.

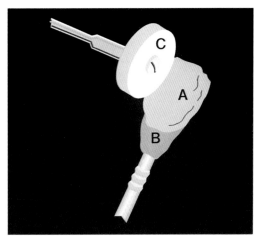

Fig 18-16 When a veneer is fabricated, the pressed core *(A)* is seated on the special die *(B)* before grinding for reduction. The veneer is much more safely manipulated in that manner; moreover, the peril of fracturing is decreased.

at a time. Investing is done in the traditional manner. At the inner side of the muffle, marks should be placed for orientation. This technique can protect the veneers against damage during devesting.

Inspection of the marginal fit of the pressed veneers. The moment the veneers are devested and have been subjected to glass bead air abrasion using low pressure, they are reseated on the die. The accuracy of the marginal adaptation should be inspected with special care by means of a magnifying glass. The IPS Empress friction paste can be used to locate areas of too much friction. Using a brush, the paste is applied to the die. The veneer is reseated, and these areas of extreme friction can be readily detected and eliminated.

Fabrication of a resin die. After adaptation of the veneers on the (gypsum) die, an additional one, made of resin, is fabricated. The color of the resin must match that of the natural tooth to be restored. This step is important because the color of the very thin veneer is easily and significantly influenced by any

underlying color. Furthermore, it serves as protective support for reduction and polishing procedures (Fig 18-16).

The reduction of a veneer means it is ground and reduced to the thickness of a natural tooth's enamel layer. If the veneer was intentionally overcontoured prior to the pressing, the entire surface must now be reduced. It is possible to reduce up to five tenths of a millimeter without endangering the veneer to fracture. The material is readily and rapidly ground using the abrasive stones and green polishing points. The cervical one third is reduced, too; it should be reduced by 1 mm as well. The layering by increments and incorporation of effects is important particularly in these areas because here we can provide a maximum of subtlety and transparency. When the reduction procedure is finished, the form of the veneer virtually equals the form of a tooth's dentin core (Figs 18-17 and 18-18).

Wash and effect bake. The veneer is steam cleaned carefully, avoiding against the slightest thermal shock. The veneer is reposi-

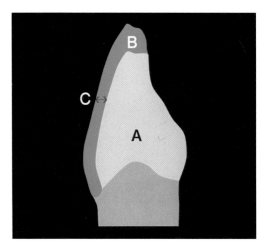

Fig 18-17 Sagittal cross section of a ceramic veneer on a natural tooth *(A)*. The thickness of the veneer can be reduced to 0.6 mm in the center *(C)*. The veneer covering the incisal third should be 1 to 1.5 mm thick *(B)*. This is the area for layering and the incorporation of effects.

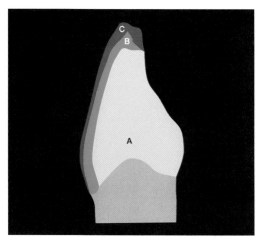

Fig 18-18 The pressed core *(B)* is reduced in order to provide space for the layering technique. This layer covers the veneer completely from the incisal region to the cervical margin. The reduction of the incisal third of a natural tooth facilitates the build-up in layers and the incorporation of effects.

tioned on the special die made of a soft resin that represents the color of the prepared natural tooth. A layer of neutral porcelain material is applied to the entire surface. Effects can be incorporated at this stage in the marginal region. If the veneer is very thin, no porcelain is applied because this could result in overcontouring; the dentin core is simply colored. These effect colors do not require space; they are applied between the dentin core and the build-up of the incisal edge. The Empress ceramic system does not require thick layers to obtain satisfactory results: tenths of a millimeter are enough to provide the material with a natural appearance (Figs 18-19 to 18-23).

Layering bake. The wash bake is performed rapidly. After the firing and the ensuing slow cooling off, no deformation will be detected, not even in the extremely thin (ie, 0.5 mm) regions. The reason for that is the difference in temperature: while the Empress core is pressed at 1,170°C, the ceramic build-up is fired at 900°C. This leaves a safety margin of 270°C, thus preventing deformation.

After each firing, the veneer must be degreased and steam cleaned. The build-up of the porcelain is also quickly performed; tenths of a millimeter provide sufficient thickness of the layer. Lateral segmentation may be used for the incisal third and new effects incorporated. One thing is important: the layer must thin out toward the finish line.

When the layering is completed and the modeling is finished, the veneer is placed on the resin die again. The contacts are slightly overcontoured and the built-up porcelain is gently condensed. Packing the particles densely can prevent detachment of the porcelain. A soft brush removes excess porcelain while the veneer remains securely seated on the die (Fig 18-24). The layer applied during the layering procedure fully

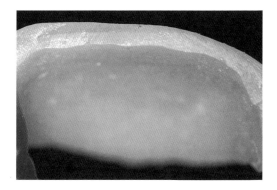

Fig 18-19 Horizontal cross section of an Empress ceramic veneer. The thickness of the veneer is 0.6 mm. Note the thin ceramic layer applied by means of the layering technique.

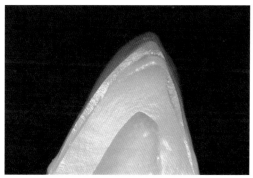

Fig 18-20 Vertical cross section of an Empress ceramic crown. Here too, as for the veneer, only a thin layer of ceramic is necessary. The layering is rapidly performed and shrinkage is virtually zero. This technique of build-up is suitable for teeth where effects are unimportant.

Fig 18-21 This section also shows the minimal thickness of the ceramic layer. It is important that the core of the pressed ceramic restoration be sufficiently thick to increase the crown's resistance to fracture.

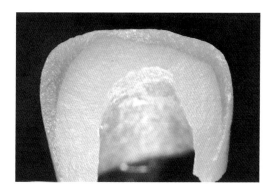

Fig 18-22 The layering is more important in this section, but the core does not suffer a decrease in strength. At times, several layers are needed to attain special effects and colors. The ceramic layers always cover the core completely.

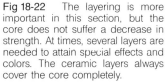

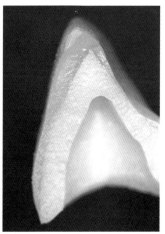

Fig 18-23 This premolar was rapidly built up, because only little space was needed for the layering. Yet it was possible to apply orange effects to the occlusal surface and to use saturated dentin porcelain for the cervical third.

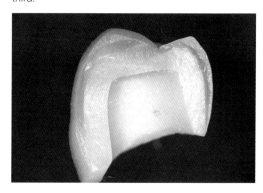

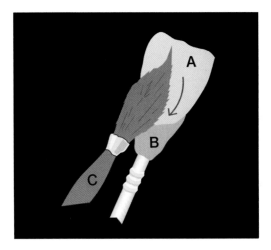

Fig 18-24 After the veneer (A) has been modeled on the working model, it is reseated on a special resin die (B). The proximal contacts are slightly overcontoured. With a very soft brush, the applied porcelain is brushed in an apical direction. The careful removal of excessive porcelain is thus readily performed down to the marginal region.

covers the veneer but thins out apically. For the firing, the veneer is placed on a nonflammable cotton-wool pad. The program of the firing cycle is as follows: drying-out for 6 minutes; heating to maximum temperature of 900°C within 60 minutes (at this temperature the vacuum is reduced for 1 minute). The firing is performed with vacuum.

Glaze bake and minimum gloss. In general, one bake suffices after the build-up; the applied porcelain is of minimum thickness. After the veneer has been removed from the furnace, shape and function are inspected as per conventional restorations. At this stage macrostructures and microstructures are established. The veneer may be additionally colored, if needed.

To perform the glaze bake, the veneer is placed on the nonflammable cotton-wool pad and put into the furnace. It is then air-fired at a temperature of 890°C (see chapter 19, "Analysis of the Surface Structure — Polish-

Fig 18-25 Completed ceramic veneers on teeth 12 to 23, 33 to 43, after polishing. The polishing is done with the veneer securely seated on the die.

Fig 18-26 Esthetic value of veneers depends mainly on the penetrability of light. The Empress ceramic core provides sufficient potential to mask discolorations without rendering the entire restoration too opaque.

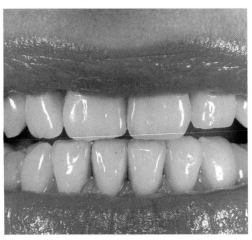

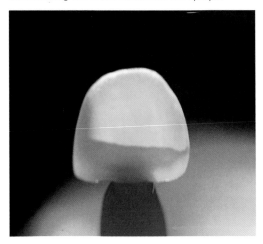

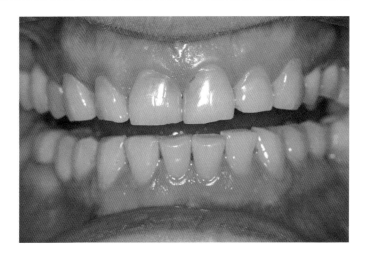

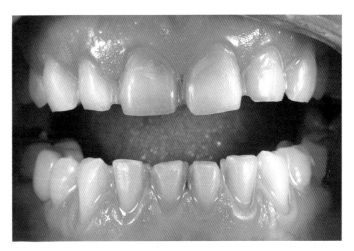

Figs 18-27 and 18-28 Preparations for 12 veneers. (Courtesy of Dr Thierry Jeannin, Orange, France).

ing"). The veneer is allowed to cool slowly after it has been recovered from the furnace. It is reseated on the resin die and polished to a high gloss (Figs 18-25 and 18-26).

This technique is simple enough to be applied in laboratory practice. Each step is traditional and certain working habits need not be changed. No fatiguing work is involved, as is the case with refractory dies. During the entire process of fabrication, color control is easy; this consequently prevents failure. Moreover, the dosage of the Empress material is perfect. It masks all discolorations with a minimum thickness of the material. Ultimately, this material exhibits great esthetic qualities, and we can mimic the appearance of a natural tooth with a thickness of only a few tenths of a millimeter (Figs 18-27 to 18-34).

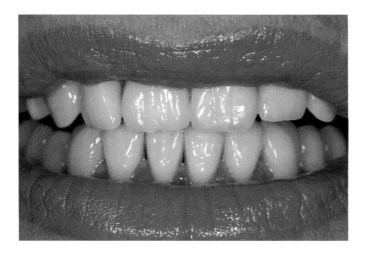

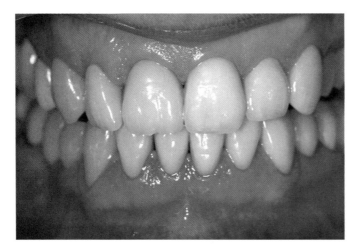

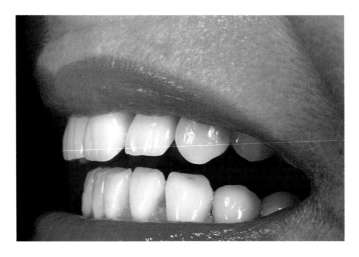

Figs 18-29 to 18-31 Empress veneers fabricated according to the layering technique. Most of them exhibit only a 0.6- to 0.8-mm-layer thickness. Note the subtle color effects in the incisal one third.

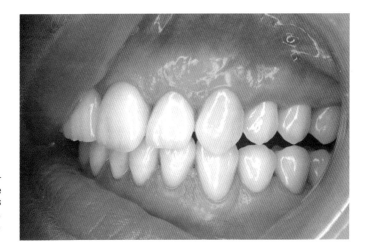

Fig 18-32 These restorations for posterior teeth on the left-hand side are made of Empress ceramic as well as metal ceramic. Teeth 24, 26, and 35: Empress ceramic. Teeth 25, 34, 36, and 37: metal ceramic.

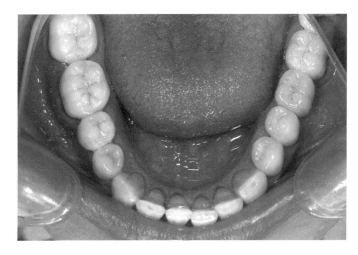

Fig 18-33 Mandibular arch viewed from above: Empress veneers on teeth 31, 32, 33, 41, 42, and 43. Empress ceramic crown on tooth 34. Porcelain inlay on tooth 44. Metal ceramic crowns on teeth 35, 36, 37, 45, 46, and 47.

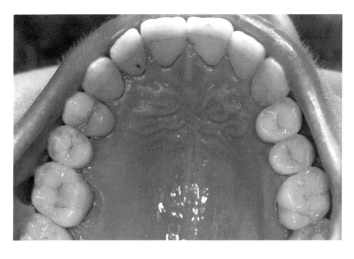

Fig 18-34 Empress veneers on teeth 21, 22, 23, 11, 12, 13, and 14. To give tooth 14 a longer appearance, the entire occlusal surface was intentionally restored in ceramic. Thus, the correct vertical dimension was reconstructed. Empres ceramic crowns on teeth 24 and 26. Metal ceramic crowns on teeth 25, 15, and 16. (Courtesy of Dr Thierry Jeannin, Orange, France.)

19 Analysis of the Surface Structure – Polishing

Polishing of porcelain is becoming an increasingly common practice in dental laboratories. It requires profound knowledge and analytic understanding of the surface structure of natural teeth as well as accurate methods.

If we carefully observe the oral cavity of a patient, it is easy to detect differences in form and symmetry between each and every tooth. A patient's smile, which apparently is very regular, reveals itself to be a mere combination of a variety of minute irregularities, malalignments, occlusal disorders – in short, a conglomerate of particularities that contribute to a natural, pleasing smile (Figs 19-1 and 19-2).

The surface structure of natural teeth, too, is made up of small irregularities, which we call macrogeography and microgeography. Light is reflected from a tooth's surface as it is from the facets of a diamond. There are distinct differences in the surface structure of teeth depending on the patient's age, position of a tooth, morphology, and even the hardness of the enamel. The surface geography of the enamel is subjected to numerous changes throughout a person's life. Therefore, it is essential to restore this macrogeography and microgeography. Consequently, the surface structure of porcelain or other cosmetic material must be adapted to the adjacent natural teeth. The successful integration of a ceramic restoration (or other cosmetic dental material) depends largely (among other reasons) on the surface structure and a well-adapted gloss.

Observation and Application of Information

Polishing of porcelain creates a natural-looking surface structure. A certain rate of attrition that took many years to develop can be achieved in a few minutes by polishing. Teeth of younger patients show numerous lines, particularly growth lines. The geography of the surface shows more complexity and less gloss (Fig 19-3). This is completely different from middle-aged or older patients: macrogeography becomes less distinct, growth lines disappear and gloss increases (Figs 19-4 and 19-5).

When the color of a restoration is communicated to the dental laboratory, the type of surface structure should always be conveyed (some lines, a few, or none at all), and gloss, too (high or low gloss, dull appearance). Gloss can be classified in degrees:

- Very glossy: 9/10 or 10/10
- Medium gloss: 7/10 or 8/10
- Little gloss: 5/10 or 6/10

If dentist and dental technician are distant from each other, this classification can help communication.

Another important medium for communication is photography. By means of a slide projector, the tooth that is to be imitated can be studied. This may lead to an exact replica of the surface structure, but characteristics, gradations, and the adjacent gingiva can be considered, too (Fig 19-6). Photography is an eminent source of information although it is much less reliable regarding color of teeth.

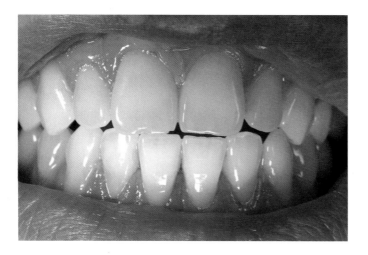

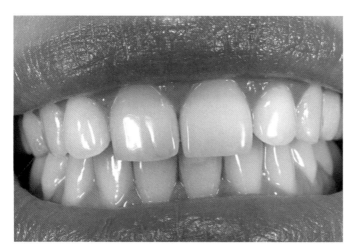

Figs 19-1 and 19-2 If patients are observed attentively when smiling, one can discern that it is not the symmetric aspects of teeth that characterize an individual smile. Small irregularities, malalignments, and different surface structures contribute significantly to a natural smile.

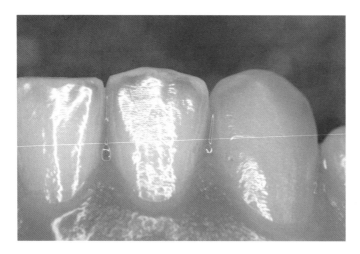

Fig 19-3 Surface structure of a young patient's teeth. Numerous growth lines and the complex geography of the surface are visible.

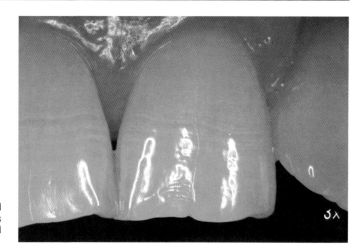

Fig 19-4 Teeth of a middle-aged patient. The macrogeography is less distinct, the growth lines vanish, and gloss increases.

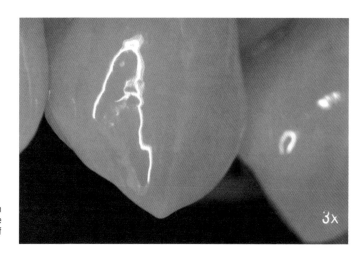

Fig 19-5 Considerable magnification facilitates thorough studies of the microgeography and the regions of light reflection.

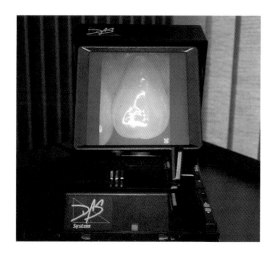

Fig 19-6 In order to improve our skill and to avoid getting lost in the maze of individual interpretation, the use of a slide projector and photographs of natural teeth can prove very helpful (D.A.S.-system, Nîmes Cedex, France).

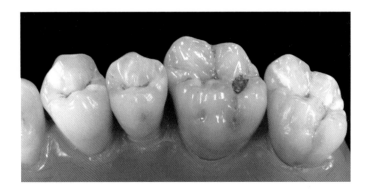

Fig 19-7 The occlusal surfaces exhibit subtle structures, too.

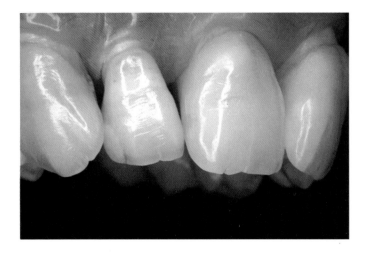

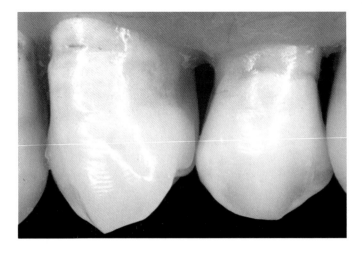

Figs 19-8 and 19-9 Study of a metal ceramic restoration. The surface structure of teeth is quite different depending on tooth position. If teeth are located in a more lingual position, they are thus more guarded, and consequently they show more lines and a matte finish. Those in a more facial position are more exposed, smoother, and exhibit more gloss.

Furthermore, it is possible to study extracted teeth and register their contour and macrogeography and microgeography.

If we try ro reconstruct the exact surface structure of the tooth to be restored, it is necessary not to neglect the occlusal surfaces (Fig 19-7). For even more accurate investigations, it is sometimes helpful to standardize teeth and place them in a study cast. The metal ceramic restorations in Figs 19-8 and 19-9 were fabricated after the surface structure had been studied thoroughly but also according to studies of color and characteristics; they are used as models. The surface structure of teeth depends on their position; if teeth are located in a more lingual position, they are more guarded, and consequently they show more lines and a matte gloss. Those in more facial position are simply more exposed, smoother, and exhibit more gloss.

This also applies to total reconstructions. The surface structure of maxillary anterior teeth is distinguished from that of mandibular teeth, which are less smooth and less glossy because they are protected by the maxilla. The maxillary central incisor in Fig 19-10 is virtually polished (an older patient), whereas

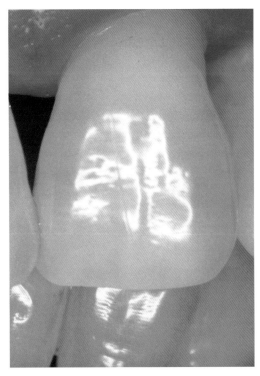

Fig 19-10   The mandibular incisors still exhibit growth lines because they are guarded against natural wear. The maxillary incisors, on the other hand, show a surface that is smoother and more glossy.

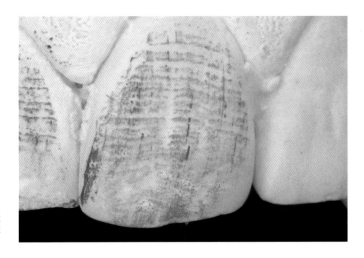

Fig 19-11 Growth lines are not always of identical appearance, but they are related to a precise pattern.

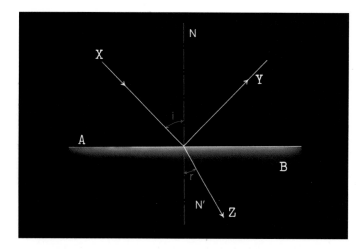

Figs 19-12 and 19-13 The reflection of light is more intense on a smooth surface than it is on a serrated one; the light rebounds.

Fig 19-12 *(X)* Light beam; *(Y)* partial reflection; *(Z)* refraction; *(A)* smooth surface; *(B)* glass pane.

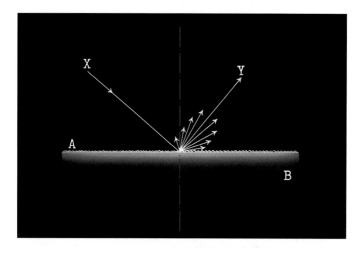

Fig 19-13 *(X)* Light beam; *(Y)* diffusion; *(A)* serrated surface; *(B)* glass pane.

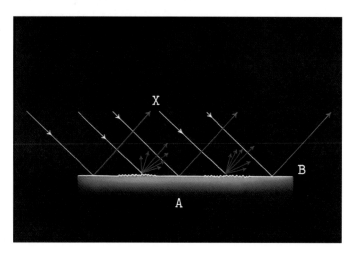

Fig 19-14 Different kinds of reflections in a certain combination on serrated *(A)* and smooth *(B)* surfaces supply a natural appearance to ceramic. *(X)* Reflection on a smooth surface; *(A)* ceramic; *(B)* surface structure.

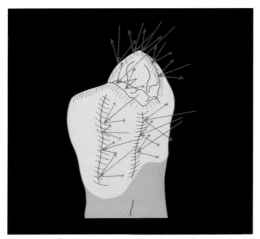

Fig 19-15 Surface structure and light reflection. Light is reflected particularly in bulging and curved areas of the teeth, which are generally very smooth.

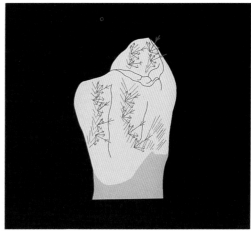

Fig 19-16 Surface structure and light reflection. In fissures and concavities, light reflection is much less significant. The result is a double light reflection between concave and convex areas.

the mandibular incisors show some growth lines. These mandibular teeth are guarded against mechanical and natural wear and therefore are not as smooth and glossy.

Growth lines are neither identical nor of the same shape or dimension (Fig 19-11); they are arranged in a precise pattern. By simply pressing articulating paper with the fingertips onto the surface of the gypsum cast, the pattern is rendered prominently.

Why should we attempt to establish a natural-appearing surface? Take the example of two fixed partial dentures, one for a younger patient, the other for an older patient. Regions that are the most prominent and, consequently, most susceptible to natural and mechanical wear, are polished to a high gloss. Concave areas that are more protected and show more growth lines are polished to a low gloss. Figures 19-12 to 19-14 illustrate clearly our objective: reflection is much more intense on a smooth surface than on a serrated surface where the light rebounds. In fact, this combination of different surface structures creates the desirable play of reflections of light (Figs 19-15 and 19-16).

After thorough studies of the macrogeography and microgeography, it is decided to incorporate growth lines into the first fixed partial denture (that for the younger patient). We draw the line pattern with a gray pencil, then we use a long, slightly tapered square-tipped diamond of medium or fine grit to recontour the growth lines. The instrument is moved tangentially to the surface, touching the porcelain over a length of 2 to 3 mm (Figs 19-17 to 19-19). We work from one side to the other with no backward motion, following the marked pattern. The lingual side is treated likewise. Articulating paper is used to inspect the result (Figs 19-20 and 19-21). When the macrogeography and microgeography are established, the concavities are polished to a low gloss. This is done by placing the work into the furnace without applying a low-fusing porcelain. The restoration can be air-fired or vacuum-fired. It may be performed during a correction bake, too. We must keep in mind, however, that we want to attain a low glaze and avoid too much firing. The final gloss should be 1/10 or 1/20 short of the maximum gloss (Fig 19-22).

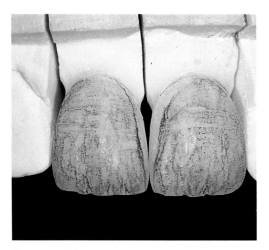

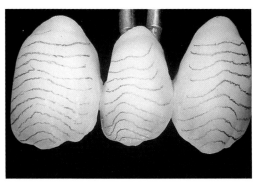

Fig 19-18 The pattern of the growth lines is marked with a pencil on the porcelain surface.

Fig 19-17 Using an pencil and articulating paper, the distinct features of the porcelain surface are marked. Shape, transition lines, and macrogeography and microgeography can be studied.

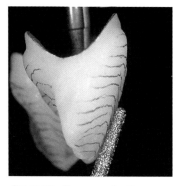

Fig 19-19 The growth lines are created mechanically with a slightly tapered round-tip diamond. The instrument is moved tangentially to the surface, touching the porcelain over a length of 2 to 3 mm.

It is difficult to specify an exact firing temperature. Ceramists neither use the same furnace or porcelain material, nor do they follow the same method of layering. This leads to different results after the firing despite identical temperatures. Also, we do not condense the porcelain. We only try to establish a low gloss that is approximately 1/10 to 1/20 below the high gloss.

As soon as the restoration is recovered from the furnace, polishing is started. Carborundum stones of the appropriate grit and shape (tapered or flame-shaped) are used for labial or lingual surfaces (Fig 19-23); carborundum disks are used for the proximal surfaces (Fig 19-24). The proximal surfaces, the cervical margin, and the underside of the restoration must be perfectly smooth to prevent plaque accumulation. A large-diameter abrasive instrument is used to finish the most exposed areas, such as protruding regions and transitions. Working at low speed on all surfaces of the restoration can create natural-looking wear. This wide grinding wheel is strictly used on convex surfaces (Fig 19-25); a smaller-diameter grinder would remove undue amounts of the surface (Fig 19-26).

After this sequence of selective polishing (in this case less important because of the

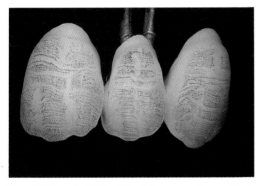 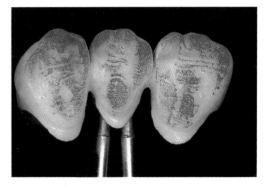

Figs 19-20 and 19-21 Articulating paper is used to inspect the growth-line pattern.

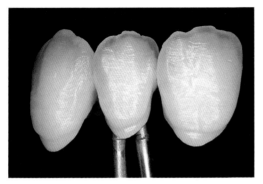

Fig 19-22 A fixed partial denture after the minimum glaze bake. This gloss should be 1/10 to 2/10 short of the maximum gloss.

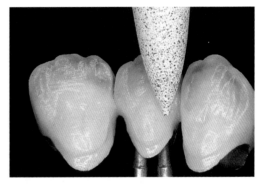

Fig 19-23 A flame-shaped abrasive stone is used for polishing. The same instrument is used for the occlusal and the lingual surfaces.

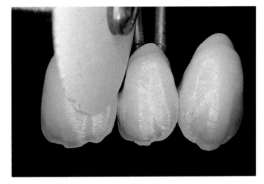

Fig 19-24 The proximal surfaces are finished with silicone disks. These surfaces must be absolutely smooth to prevent plaque accumulation.

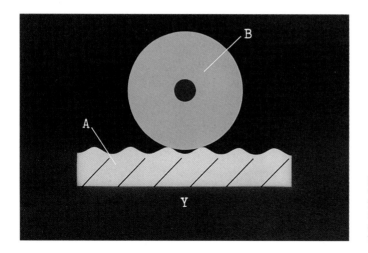

Fig 19-25 Wide silicone and felt wheels are used on all convex surfaces. *(A)* Porcelain; *(B)* large-diameter felt wheel, diamond paste; *(Y)* convex surfaces show more gloss than concave ones.

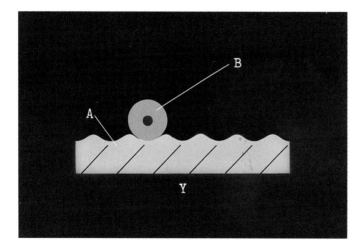

Fig 19-26 An abrasive wheel of smaller diameter would polish not only the convex surfaces but the concave ones, too. Thus, we obtain neither the desired double reflection nor the double gloss. *(A)* Ceramic; *(B)* small-diameter felt wheel with diamond paste; *(Y)* the concave and the convex surfaces will show equal gloss.

patient's youth), the high gloss is attained. We use identically shaped felt polishers in combination with high-quality diamond paste (Fig 19-27). Polishing of the desired surfaces creates more gloss, and more reflection as well, on convex surfaces. Ultimately, this will result in a magnificent play of light between these two levels of gloss. Light on a porcelain surface acts in the same way as on natural teeth (Fig 19-28). If a traditional glaze bake were performed, this play of light reflections would not exist: the degree of gloss between concave and convex areas would be identical.

If a fixed partial denture for an older patient is to be fabricated, the polishing sequence is even more important because we have to consider a greater number of smooth surfaces. The following instruments should be used to design the macrogeography and microgeography:

- A flame-shaped, tapered diamond is used to form depressions (ie, small concavities); the same instrument can be used on the interproximal space (Fig 19-29).
- An inverted cone diamond is used to recontour lines or emphasize the cemen-

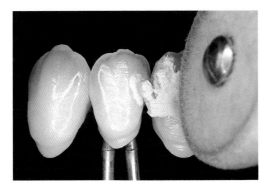

Fig 19-27 Polishing of the ceramic with felt wheel and diamond polishing paste in order to give the restoration a high gloss. The diamond paste should be white and have a fine grain to avoid contamination and roughening of the porcelain.

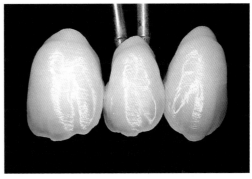

Fig 19-28 Completed restoration. The light acts on the ceramic just as on the surface of natural teeth.

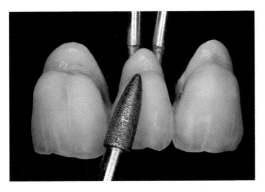

Fig 19-29 Fixed partial denture for an older patient. Treatment of the surface with a flame-shaped diamond creates the macrogeography.

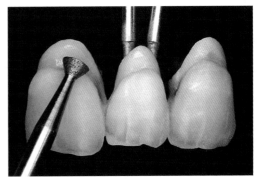

Fig 19-30 An inverted cone diamond is used to recontour lines or emphasize the cementoenamel junction of the restoration.

toenamel junction of the restoration (Fig 19-30).

For reasons of accuracy, a magnifying glass should always be used. Photographs, considerably magnified, are of great help. The restoration is now placed in the furnace in order to create a low gloss (glazing of the concave surfaces). Polishing can then be done using abrasive stones. This procedure is very important because restored teeth for older patients must have smoother surfaces (Figs 19-31 to 19-33). The proximal and cervical surfaces and the underside of the

restoration are polished. The same procedure is performed to create a high gloss, with diamond paste and felt polisher used at a slightly higher speed (Figs 19-34 and 19-35).

The finished restoration will exhibit a satisfying play of light reflection (Fig 19-36). These surfaces, which are very smooth in prominent areas, prove the high esthetic quality of porcelain. It is necessary to use fine-grain porcelain. (IPS Ivoclar has reduced the grain size by 23%.) This refined powder facilitates the modeling of fine surface structures and provides the restoration with higher stability

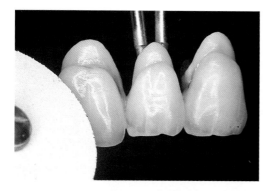

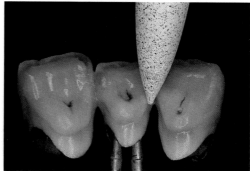

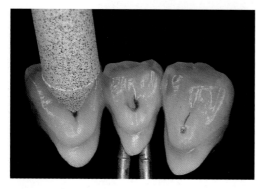

Figs 19-31 to 19-33 The porcelain surfaces are polished after the minimum glaze bake with a variety of abrasive silicone points. This restoration for an older patient requires even more polishing.

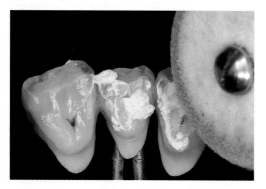

Figs 19-34 and 19-35 A high gloss is achieved with diamond polishing paste and felt polishers (felt wheel or flame-shaped, depending on the surface).

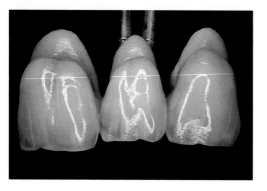

Fig 19-36 The finished restoration and the "play of double light reflection": a low gloss on the concave and a high gloss on the convex surfaces.

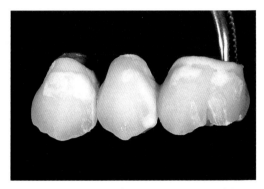 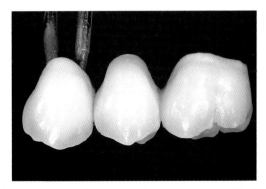

Figs 19-37 and 19-38 Correction bake and minimum glaze bake are carried out simultaneously (vacuum-firing). When the restoration is recovered from the furnace, only the corrected areas need to be repolished and a high gloss must be achieved.

but less shrinkage and brittleness. The entire coloration is created inside the porcelain itself according to the layering technique and lateral segmentation.

Finally, we would like to emphasize the advantage of performing two firings. Figures 19-37 and 19-38 showe that a correction bake and a minimum glaze bake can be carried out simultaneously (vacuum-firing in this case). This is enormously time-saving compared to the traditional method of performing correction and glaze bakes separately.

As can be seen in Figs 19-39 and 19-40, the surface structure of the metal ceramic restoration on tooth 11 is not of satisfactory quality. During the trial seating procedure, poor light reflection was noticeable. After corrective polishing, this crown fits considerably better

into the dental arch because of improved light reflection. This example emphasizes the significance of gloss and quality of surface structure. It is less detrimental to misjudge the hue by one quarter than to give the restoration a poor surface structure.

In conclusion, the key words for successful mimicking of surface structure are observation, high and low gloss and, in addition, the play of light reflection. Instruments that are appropriate as well as efficient make the objective simpler and more comfortable, rendering any additional manipulation redundant. These instruments (together with the technique) are available in a kit standardized by the author (Fig 19-41): the selected instruments are coordinated according to their grain size.

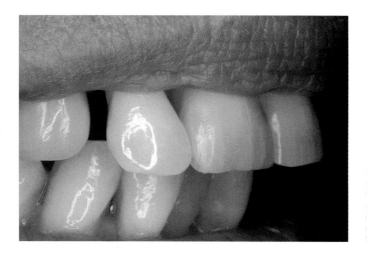

Fig 19-39 Tooth 11 is restored with a metal ceramic crown, the surface structure and degree of gloss are unsatisfactory. The restoration is conspicuous because of the discrepancy in light reflection to natural teeth.

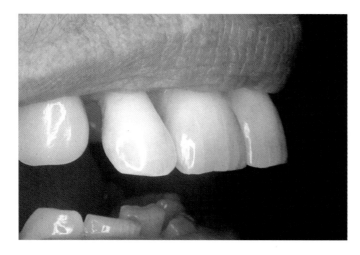

Fig 19-40 After corrective polishing and glazing, it is possible to integrate the crown into the dental arch. This example clearly shows the significance of surface structure.

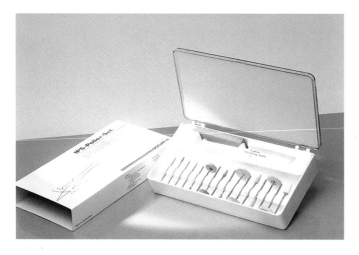

Fig 19-41 The polishing kit by Ivoclar, small version.

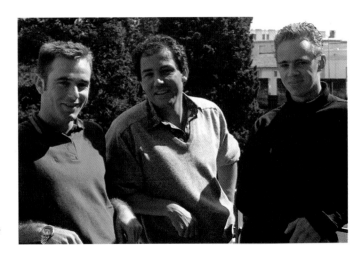

My two colleagues, *Jean-Marie Milesi* and *Jean-François Zalejski.*

This work would be most incomplete without emphasizing strongly the significance of a team whose contributions are absolutely indispensable in the quest for naturalness, function, and accuracy. Therefore, our leitmotif must be: to question the achieved day in, day out, in order to go beyond our possibilities and knowledge.

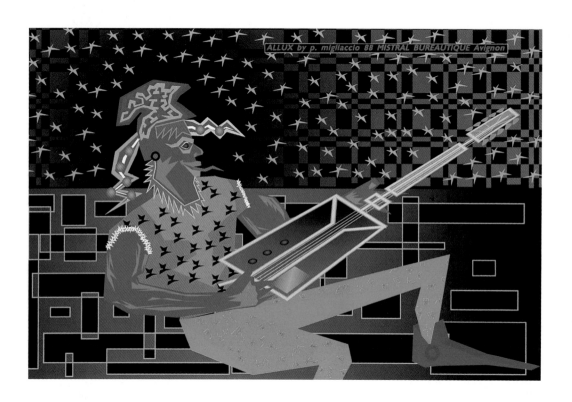

References

Abendroth U. Das Herstellen von Kronen aus gießbarer Dicorglaskeramik. Dent Labor 1985; 33: 1281 – 1286.

Adair PJ. Dental constructs and tools and production thereof. EP 00 22655. 1986.

Adair PJ, Grossman DG. The castable ceramic crown. Int J Periodont Rest Dent 1984; 4: 33 – 45.

Allard Y. L'Empress: Une Nouvelle Céramique Sans Armature [thesis]. Lyon: University of Lyon.

Anusavice KJ. Stress distribution in atypical crown designs. In: *Preston JD* (ed). Perspectives in Dental Ceramics: Proceedings of the Fourth International Symposium on Ceramics. Chicago: Quintessence, 1988: 175 – 191.

ASTM, Kartei: ICPDS 15 – 47. Philadelphia: American Society for Testing Material.

Barreiro MM. Phase identification in dental porcelains for ceramo-metallic restorations. Dent Mater 1989; 5: 51 – 57.

Beham G. Recherche et développement [Report No. 6]. Schaan: Département de la Prothèse, 1990.

Böttger, H, Rosenbauer KA, Pospiech P. Vergleichende rasterelektronenmikroskopische Randspaltmessungen von verblendeten und unverblendeten Metallkronen und Dicorglaskeramikkronen. Zahnärztl Welt 1988; 95: 445 – 450.

Bourelly G, Prasad A. Le procédé Optec HSP Concepts et mise en œuvre au Laboratoirc. Cahiers Prothèse 1989; 68.

Bowen KH. Moderne keramische Werkstoffe. Spektrum Wissenschaft 1986; 12: 140 – 149.

Cavel WT, Kelsey WP III, Barkmeier WW, Blankenau RJ. A pilot study of the clinical evaluation of castable ceramic inlays and a dual-cure resin cement. Quintessence Int 1988; 19: 257 – 262.

Chiche GJ, Pinault A. Essentials of Dental Ceramics: An Artistic Approach. Chicago: Year Book, 1988.

Rouffignac M de, Cooman J. Reconstitution céramométalliques des dents dépulpées destinées à recevoir des coiffes sans alliage. RFPD Actualités 1990 Nov; 21.

Dubois de Chemant N. Sur les advantages des nouvelles dents et rateliers arteficiels, incorruptables et sans odeur. London et Paris, 1788.

Glocker R. Materialprüfung mit Röntgenstrahlen. Berlin: Springer Verlag, 1958.

Grossmann DG. Tetrasilic mica glass ceramic method, US patent 3,732,087. 1973.

Hegenbarth EA. Creative Ceramic Color: A Practical System. Chicago: Quintessence, 1989.

Itten J. Art de la Couleur. Paris: Editions Dessair et Tolra, 1967.

Kedge M. Lateral, segmental buildup. In: *Preston JD* (ed). Perspectives in Dental Ceramics: Proceedings of the Fourth International Symposium on Ceramics. Chicago: Quintessence, 1988: 369 – 373.

Klug HP. X-ray Diffraction Procedures for Polycrystalline and Amorphoium Materials. New York: John Wiley and Sons.

Knellessen C, Degrange M. Les inlays onlays en vitrocéramique vers une nouvelle forme de dentisterie restauratrice. Cahiers Prothèse 1987; 60.

Kuwata M. Theory and Practice for Ceramo Metal Restorations. Chicago: Quintessence, 1980.

Lejoyeux J. Prothèse Complète Tome 2, ed 4. Paris: Editions Maloine, 1986.

Mac Culloch WT. Advances in dental ceramics. Brit Dent J 1968; 123: 361 – 365.

Mackert JR. Effects of thermally induced changes on porcelain-metal compatibility. In: Preston JD (ed). Perspectives in Dental Ceramics: Proceedings of the Fourth International Symposium on Ceramics. Chicago: Quintessence, 1988: 53 – 64.

Muia PJ. The Four Dimensional Tooth Color System. Chicago: Quintessence, 1982.

Müterthies K. Esthetic Approach to Metal Ceramic Restorations for the Mandibular Anterior Region. London: Quintessence, 1990.

N. N. Verfahren zur Herstellung von Gegenständen aus Porzellan und dgl. Patentschrift 157210. Deutsches Reich, 1937.

Parramon J-M. La Couleur et le Peintre. Paris: Editions Bordas, 1985.

Pichard C. Infrastructure ajourée. Cahiers Prothèse 1982; 40.

Prasad A, Day GP, Tobey RG. A new dimension for evaluation of porcelain-alloy compatibility. In: *Preston JD* (ed). Perspectives in Dental Ceramics: Proceedings of the Fourth International Symposium on Ceramics. Chicago: Quintessence, 1988: 65 – 74.

Roge M, Preston JD. Couleur, lumière et perception de la forme. Odontologia 1987; Dec: 357 – 362.

Shillingburg HT, Jacobi R, Brackett SE. Fundamentals of Tooth Preparations for Cast Metal and Porcelain Restorations. Chicago: Quintessence, 1987.

Simon J, Feuillerat B, Rivoire G, Kraft J-L. Le polissage technique de finition des éléments céramiques. Cahiers Prothèse 1987; 60.

Soom U. Glaskeramik. Spezialanwendung: nichtmetallische gegossene Füllungen im Seitenzahnbereich. Schweiz Mschr Zahnheilk 1987; 97: 1409 – 1416.

Stookey SD. Catalyzed crystallization of glass in theory and practice. Glastechn Ber 1959; 32 K: 1 – 8.

Touati B, Bersay L. Emaillage des dents au moyen de facettes de vitrocéramique. Cahiers Prothèse 1987; 60.

Touati B. Le collage des inlays onlays de céramique. Rev Odont Stomatol 1988; 1.

Touati B, Pissis P. L'inlay collé en résine composite. Cahiers Prothèse 1984; 48.

Touati B, Pissis P, Miara P. Restaurations unitaires collées et concept des préparations pelliculaires. Cahiers Prothèse 1985; 52.

Ubassy G. Analyse der anatomischen Oberflächenbeschaffenheit. Dent Labor 1990; 4: 493.

Ubassy G. Les Cires Colorées. RFPD Actualités 1989; 2.

Ubassy G. Les fêlures d'émail. Prothèse Dent 1989; 31: 7.

Vidal R, Dejou J, Deyez O. Les onlays de céramique conventionelle, une solution esthétique durable. Cahiers Prothèse 1987; 60.

Vogel W. Struktur und Kristallisation der Gläser. Leipzig: VEB Deutscher Verlag für Grundstoff-Industrie, 1971.

Wohlwend A, Strub JR, Schärer P. Metal ceramic and all-porcelain restorations: current considerations. Int J Prosthodont 1989; 2: 13 – 26.

Wohlwend A. Verfahren und Ofen zur Herstellung von Zahnersatzteilen. Europäische Patentanmeldung 0231 773. 1987.

Yamamoto M. Metal-Ceramics: Principles and Methods of Makoto Yamamoto. Chicago: Quintessence, 1985.

Index